Y0-ABU-323

Cardiology

Pearls & Pitfalls

VOLUME 2

Diagnosing hypertension

Editor
Joel M. Neutel, MD

Target audience
Cardiologists

Goals of this activity are to provide better understanding of the signs and symptoms of hypertension, to identify its possible underlying causes and sequelae, and to ensure accurate and rapid diagnosis and treatment.

 Scientific Exchange Inc. is accredited by the Accreditation Council for Continuing Medical Education to sponsor continuing medical education for physicians.

This activity was released on September 1, 1998. It was planned and produced in accordance with the ACCME Essentials.

Credit

Scientific Exchange Inc. designates this educational activity for a maximum of 1.5 hours in category 1 credit toward the AMA Physician's Recognition Award. Each physician should claim only those hours of credit that he or she actually spent in the educational activity.

To receive credit, you must:

1. Study this monograph.
2. Record your answers (page 76) to the self-assessment questions that follow each case study, and complete the evaluation form (pages 73-74). Return as indicated on the CME registration form (page 75).

Release date: September 1, 1998.
Expiration: Credit will be awarded for required materials postmarked or received no later than December 31, 1999. A CME certificate will be mailed within 4 to 6 weeks. No refunds will be made.

Nonphysicians

Participants who are not physicians and who complete and submit the self-assessment and evaluation questions and registration form will be sent a certificate of participation within 4 to 6 weeks.

Front cover courtesy of the National Library of Medicine.

Editor

Joel M. Neutel, MD
Assistant Clinical Professor of Medicine
University of California, Irvine, College of Medicine
Chief, Section of Clinical Pharmacology and Hypertension
Veterans Affairs Medical Center
Long Beach, California

Contributing authors

Prakash C. Deedwania, MD
Clinical Professor of Medicine
Stanford University
    School of Medicine
Stanford, California
Chief of Cardiology Division
University of California,
    San Francisco
School of Medicine

Brian D. Hoit, MD
Professor of Medicine
Division of Cardiology
University of Cincinnati
    College of Medicine
Cincinnati, Ohio

Jennifer Kaseta, MD
Research Fellow
Division of Endocrinology,
    Metabolism,
    and Hypertension
Wayne State University
    School of Medicine
Detroit, Michigan

Rene A. Oliveros, MD
Heart and Vascular Institute
San Antonio, Texas

L. Michael Prisant, MD
Professor of Medicine
Department of Medicine
Section of Cardiology
Medical College of Georgia
Augusta, Georgia

James R. Sowers, MD
Professor of Medicine
    and Physiology
Director, Division of
    Endocrinology,
    Metabolism,
    and Hypertension
Wayne State University
    School of Medicine
Detroit, Michigan

Matthew R. Weir, MD
Professor and Director
Division of Nephrology
    & Clinical Research Unit
University of Maryland
    School of Medicine
Baltimore, Maryland

Program director

Gregory Scott, PharmD
Director of Continuing Education
Scientific Exchange Inc.
(203) 618-4300

Disclosure

Disclaimer

Financial support

This activity is supported by an unrestricted educational grant
from Bristol-Myers Squibb.

Learning objectives

After completing this CME activity, cardiologists should be better able to:

1. Recognize the signs and symptoms of hypertension.

2. Describe the roles of the history, physical examination, and laboratory evaluation in diagnosing hypertension.

3. Identify the steps required to reliably detect hypertension.

4. Define the underlying causes of hypertension.

5. Distinguish and manage the sequelae of hypertension.

Contents

Hypertension:
A familiar—yet often overlooked—diagnosis

Hypertension has been and remains one of the most widely studied disorders in the field of medicine. Countless nonpharmacologic and pharmacologic measures have been and are being developed to prevent the varied complications of this disease.

Despite great advances in the understanding and treatment of hypertension, the diagnosis is missed in a significant percentage of patients. Explanations for this are numerous and range from patient denial to imprecise blood pressure (BP) monitoring. In many other instances, hypertension is recognized, but secondary causes are overlooked.

This *Pearls and Pitfalls,* the second volume in a three-volume series, presents cases relevant to the diagnosis of hypertension. Volume 1 addresses the epidemiology and pathophysiology of the disorder; volume 3 focuses on treatment. We have designed this volume to help busy practitioners recognize clinical clues forewarning that a more critical problem than essential hypertension could be the cause of a patient's elevated BP.

We hope that you enjoy this selection of case studies and that you discover some clinical pearls that will be of use to you in your everyday practice.

Joel M. Neutel, MD
Editor

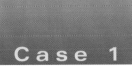

MULTIPLE CARDIOVASCULAR RISK FACTORS IN A 40-YEAR-OLD MAN

Patient presentation

A 40-year-old white man comes to the office for a routine physical examination. He has a 1-year history of mild hypertension. At the encouragement of his physician, he has tried to increase his exercise, to lose weight, and to reduce his alcohol and salt intake. The patient has no other medical problems. He is an accountant, and he admits that his only exercise is an occasional game of golf. He is a nonsmoker, and he is currently taking no medication. His father, who also has a history of hypertension, had a myocardial infarction at the age of 52 years.

Physical examination

Physical examination findings reveal: height, 5 ft 10 in; weight, 240 lb; blood pressure (BP), 158/94 mm Hg; pulse, 78 beats per minute. The patient is normocephalic without injury. Extraocular movements are full, and the pupils are equal and reactive to light. Funduscopic examination is normal. The lungs are clear. The S_1 and S_2 are normal, but no S_3 or S_4 is present. There are no murmurs. The abdomen is soft and nontender. There is no organomegaly. Bowel sounds are normal. There is no peripheral edema in the extremities; peripheral pulses are full and easily palpated. There is no cyanosis, jaundice, or clubbing. The central nervous system is grossly intact.

Laboratory evaluation

Laboratory tests show the following levels: blood urea nitrogen, 24 mg/dL; creatinine, 0.9 mg/dL; total cholesterol, 248 mg/dL; low-density lipoprotein cholesterol, 156 mg/dL; and glucose, 136 mg/dL. Electrocardiograph shows normal sinus rhythm and axis and is in normal limits.

Questions

What is the optimal treatment for this patient's high blood pressure?

What other risk factors should be approached in the management of this patient?

Discussion and management

Mild hypertension is often treated conservatively. In this case, however, the patient also has slightly elevated cholesterol levels and borderline, diet-controlled diabetes. Moreover, he has other cardiovascular risk factors: obesity, a sedentary lifestyle, and a family history of cardiovascular disease. Addressed individually, these risk factors are mild and would also be treated conservatively. But when such risk factors occur together, they act synergistically, and cardiovascular disease may result. Consequently, because this patient is at significantly increased risk for cardiovascular disease, his risk factors should be managed aggressively.

Early pharmacologic treatment of this patient's mild hypertension and mild hypercholesterolemia and modification of his lifestyle are warranted. Although it is important that he lose weight and exercise, his attempts to do so over the last year have been unsuccessful. If in his current efforts, he succeeds in losing weight, in maintaining an improved exercise program, and in reducing his alcohol and salt intake for 6 months or longer, pharmacologic treatment may be discontinued for a trial period. Few patients achieve and maintain such success, however.

While diet control of his borderline diabetes may be appropriate for now, his condition must be closely monitored. If careful adherence to his diet fails to control his diabetes, drug treatment will have to be considered. Early treatment of such patients affords them protection, most likely with decreased cardiovascular risk. Drugs that block the renin-angiotensin system—angiotensin receptor blockers (ARBs) and angiotensin-converting enzyme inhibitors—will frequently reduce BP and other cardiovascular risk factors. If pharmacologic treatment becomes necessary for this patient, an ARB will be an ideal choice.

CLINICAL PEARLS AND PITFALLS

- Multiple risk factors, although individually mild, should be treated aggressively when they occur together.

- In such patients, it is best to begin drug treatment early and to encourage lifestyle modification. If patients are successful in losing weight, maintaining exercise, and reducing salt and alcohol intake, antihypertensive treatment may be discontinued for a trial period.

- Cardiovascular risk factors synergistically cause heart disease.

Additional reading

Assmann G, Cullen P, Schulte H. The Munster Heart Study (PROCAM). Results of follow-up at 8 years. *Eur Heart J.* 1998;19(suppl A):A2-A11.

Lindahl B, Nilsson TK, Asplund K, et al. Intense nonpharmacological intervention in subjects with multiple cardiovascular risk factors: Decreased fasting insulin levels but only a minor effect on plasma plasminogen activator inhibitor activity. *Metabolism.* 1998;47:384-390.

Case 1. Self-assessment questions

1. Mild hypertension, moderately high cholesterol levels, and borderline diabetes present concurrently should be treated conservatively with minimal medical intervention.
   a. True   b. False

2. In most patients, treating hypertension nonpharmacologically successfully controls blood pressure (BP).
   a. True   b. False

3. _____ is the drug of choice for control of BP in a patient with diabetes mellitus.
   a. An angiotensin-converting enzyme (ACE) inhibitor
   b. A β-blocker
   c. A diuretic
   d. An angiotensin receptor blocker (ARB)

4. ARBs and ACE inhibitors will frequently reduce BP and other cardiovascular risk factors.
   a. True   b. False

Answer form on page 76.

ABNORMAL CHEST FILM AND LEG PAIN IN A TEENAGER

Patient presentation

A 16-year-old white male is evaluated for an abnormal chest film. The patient does not complain of any symptoms but says that exercise causes discomfort in his legs. Consequently, he cannot participate in sports.

Physical examination

Physical examination shows a well-developed young man with a normal body habitus. He is in no acute distress. Vital signs are: blood pressure (BP), 180/90 mm Hg in both arms; pulse, 84 beats per minute. Respirations are normal. Fundi are normal, as is the jugular venous pulse. Carotid and brachial pulses are bounding and have a rapid rise. A thrill is evident in the suprasternal notch. The lungs are clear to percussion and auscultation.

Cardiac examination shows that the left ventricle is slightly displaced. S_1 is normal, S_2 is accentuated, and an S_4 is present. A grade 2/6 midsystolic murmur is heard over the anterior precordium and posterior thorax. An abdominal examination is unremarkable, without masses or bruits. Femoral pulses are markedly decreased and delayed compared with brachial pulses. There is no cyanosis, clubbing, or edema.

Laboratory evaluation

Electrocardiogram reveals left ventricular hypertrophy. A chest film shows a bulge that resembles the numeral three and is located above and below the aortic knob, notching of the ribs over their inferior margin, and mild left ventricular enlargement.

Questions

What is the cause of hypertension in this patient?

What is the prognosis?

How would it be best to evaluate this abnormality?

How should this patient be managed?

Discussion and management

Secondary hypertension, as evidenced in this case, may result from any of a diverse group of disorders. The Sixth Report of the Joint National Committee on Prevention, Detection, Evaluation, and Treatment of High Blood Pressure recommends investigating possible causes when the index of suspicion is high.[1] Clues such as sudden onset of hypertension, severe hypertension, or a poor or altered response to therapy can suggest a specific underlying problem.

Common causes of secondary hypertension include oral contraceptive use, renal parenchymal disease (indicated by enlarged kidneys, increased serum creatinine levels, abnormalities on urinalysis), and renovascular disease (abdominal bruits). A few cases result from endocrine disorders, such as primary hyperaldosteronism (unprovoked hypokalemia), Cushing's syndrome (truncal obesity, purple striae), hyperparathyroidism (unprovoked hypercalcemia), pheochromocytoma (labile BP, headache, palpitations, pallor), and coarctation of the aorta.

Coarctation, or congenital narrowing, of the aorta is the cause of hypertension in the patient in this case. Coarctation is usually—but not invariably—just distal to the left subclavian artery. Cardiac lesions, such as bicuspid aortic valve, patent ductus arteriosus, or a ventricular septal defect, may be associated. Such lesions, combined with the severity and rapidity of obstruction, are important in determining the age at which the patient presents and the natural history of the coarctation.

Symptoms of coarctation may occur in early infancy, but some patients do not present until the second or third decade of life. Nearly all affected show symptoms and complications by the age of 40 years. Survival beyond 50 years is unusual.

Interestingly, mechanical obstruction is not the cause of hypertension in coarctation. Rather, elevated BP results from poorly understood mechanisms that involve stimulation of the sympathetic nervous system and renin-angiotensin system. In uncorrected cases, the associated hypertension may lead to left ventricular failure and premature coronary artery disease—the most common cause of death in affected patients.

Clinical findings prompt the suspicion of coarctation. On physical examination, the hallmark of the disorder is upper extremity hypertension with weak and delayed or absent femoral pulses. Radiographic evidence of prestenotic and poststenotic aortic dilatation and rib notching, due to dilated collaterals originating in the subclavian artery, confirms the diagnosis.

Doppler echocardiography supersedes barium esophagography as the evaluation technique of choice (Figure 1). Two-dimensional echocardiographic imaging from several views (suprasternal, high parasternal, subcostal) is useful in defining the narrowed aorta,[2] and Doppler velocimetry helps in estimating the peak instantaneous gradient when using the modified Bernoulli equation. Associated lesions are also readily identified.

Coarctation may be managed medically, with treatment aimed at associated cardiovascular abnormalities; prophylactically, with lifelong protection against endocarditis; or surgically, with resection and end-to-end anastomosis in patients 3-5 years of age. Primary repair using percutaneous balloon angioplasty can cause problems, due to residual gradients and the potential for iatrogenic aortic disease (aneurysm, dissection, rupture). Angioplasty has a clear role in the treatment of recoarctation, however.[3]

After childhood, surgery often results in residual hypertension—or paradoxical hypertension—despite the relief of obstruction.[4,5] The severity of hypertension correlates with the duration of presurgical hypertension. Paradoxical hypertension is best prevented and treated with β-blockers. Following surgery, risks associated with infective endocarditis, stroke, and aortic dissection persist and warrant careful management.

In this case, the patient had successful surgery, with no residual coarctation on follow-up Doppler study. A week before undergoing the procedure, the patient was given β-blockers. The agents were continued afterward for mild postoperative hypertension.

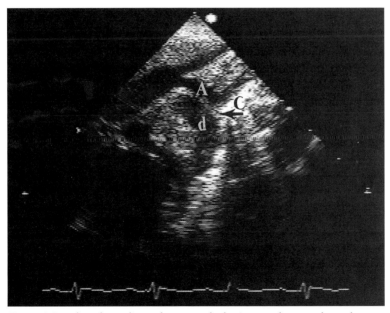

Figure 1. Doppler echocardiography supersedes barium esophagography as the diagnostic technique of choice. Two-dimensional imaging from several views (suprasternal, high parasternal, subcostal) is useful in defining the narrowed aorta (A). This two-dimensional echocardiogram (suprasternal notch view) clearly shows the ductus (d), which has been pharmacologically dilated. The arrow indicates coarctation (C).

CLINICAL PEARLS AND PITFALLS

- Among the most common causes of secondary hypertension are oral contraceptive use, renal parenchymal disease, and renovascular disease.
- Upper extremity hypertension with weak and delayed or absent femoral pulses is the hallmark of coarctation of the aorta.
- Doppler echocardiography is the initial evaluation technique of choice.

References

1. The Sixth Report of the Joint National Committee on Prevention, Detection, Evaluation, and Treatment of High Blood Pressure. *Arch Intern Med.* 1997;157:243-244.
2. George B, DiSessa TG, Williams R, et al. Coarctation repair without cardiac catheterization in infants. *Am Heart J.* 1987;114:1421-1425.
3. Choy M, Rocchini AP, Beekman RH, et al. Paradoxical hypertension after repair of coarctation of the aorta in children: Balloon angioplasty versus surgical repair. *Circulation.* 1987;75:1186-1191.
4. Murphy AM, Blades M, Daniels S, et al. Blood pressure and cardiac output during exercise: A longitudinal study of children undergoing repair of coarctation. *Am Heart J.* 1989;117:1327-1332.
5. Cohen M, Fuster V, Steele PM, et al. Coarctation of the aorta. Long-term follow-up and prediction of outcome after surgical correction. *Circulation.* 1989;80:840-845.

Case 2. Self-assessment questions

1. Among the most common causes of secondary hypertension are _____.
   a. oral contraceptive use
   b. renal parenchymal disease
   c. renovascular disease
   d. coarctation of the aorta
   e. a, b, and c

2. The hallmark of coarctation of the aorta is upper extremity hypertension with weak and delayed or absent femoral pulses.
   a. True   b. False

3. Radiographic evidence of prestenotic and poststenotic aortic dilatation and rib notching confirms the diagnosis of coarctation of the aorta.
   a. True   b. False

4. Hypertension in coarctation results from mechanical obstruction.
   a. True   b. False

Answer form on page 76.

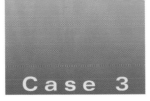

HEADACHE AND BLURRED VISION
IN A 36-YEAR-OLD WHITE WOMAN

Patient presentation

A 36-year-old unemployed white woman comes to the emergency department and complains of headache and blurred vision. Her boyfriend says that over the last 6 hours, she has become confused and nauseous and has vomited. She denies any head trauma. Although she admits to cocaine use in the past, she says she has not taken the drug in 3 years. Her current medications are birth control pills, over-the-counter sinus tablets, and ibuprofen for sinus headaches. She smokes one pack of cigarettes per day. Her only hospitalization was during a pregnancy when she was 18 years old. Early in the pregnancy and at follow-up, her blood pressure (BP) was elevated, but she has not visited any physician since that time.

Physical examination

Vital signs are: BP, 220/146 mm Hg; pulse, 98 beats per minute; respiration, 32 breaths per minute. Height, 5 ft 4 in; weight, 130 lb. There is no icterus. Figure 1 shows funduscopic findings. There is no jugular venous distention at 30° or carotid bruits. The thyroid gland is unremarkable. The lungs are clear without rales or wheezes. The left ventricular apical impulse is displaced outside the midclavicular line, enlarged in diameter and sustained. The cardiac rhythm is regular. The S_1 is within normal limits, and the S_2 is split physiologically. There is a loud S_4, but no S_3 gallop or murmur.

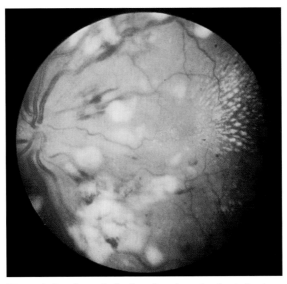

Figure 1. Funduscopic findings in a hypertensive patient with headache and blurred vision.

Abdominal examination is unremarkable, without bruits. No femoral bruits are auscultated. Peripheral pulses are 2+ and equal in the upper and lower extremities without any clubbing, cyanosis, or edema. Neurologic examination does not suggest focal abnormalities. There is no nuchal rigidity.

Laboratory evaluation

Laboratory findings show the following levels: blood urea nitrogen, 44 mg/dL; creatinine, 3.1 mg/dL; potassium, 3.2 mEq/dL; uric acid, 9.8 mg/dL. A complete blood cell count shows mildly increased reticulocytes, and helmet cells are reported on the peripheral smear. Urinalysis demonstrates red blood cell casts and red blood cells. Urine drug screen is negative. An electrocardiogram shows increased voltage. Computed tomography scan does not show any focal abnormalities.

Questions

Who is at risk for a hypertensive emergency?

What diagnostic clues should be noted?

Discussion and management

Although hypertensive emergencies are less common now than they were in the past, they still occur. Such emergencies are more likely to develop in patients who smoke, who are noncompliant, who are indigent, who are African American, and who take oral contraceptives. Characteristics of a hypertensive emergency include a diastolic BP that is usually higher than 140 mm Hg (Table 1).

TABLE 1
Characteristics of hypertensive emergency

- Diastolic blood pressure usually higher than 140 mm Hg
- Congestive heart failure, cardiac enlargement, prominent apical impulse
- Funduscopic evidence of hemorrhages, exudates, papilledema
- Headache, confusion, somnolence, stupor, visual loss, focal deficits, seizures, coma
- Nausea, vomiting
- Oliguria, azotemia

The differential diagnosis includes secondary hypertension, resulting from such disorders as renovascular disease, pheochromocytoma, and primary aldosteronism (Table 2). Other conditions may also mimic hypertensive crisis.

Key physical findings of hypertensive emergency include retinal flame-shaped hemorrhages, cotton-wool spots, and papilledema. Other important clues, such as hematuria, red blood cell casts, progressive azotemia, myocardial ischemia, heart failure, and intravascular hemolysis, also suggest the condition. Visual complaints, nausea, vomiting, altered mental status, and headaches could indicate hypertensive encephalopathy. Seizures and focal neurologic findings may also be present.

High levels of angiotensin II, norepinephrine, and other vasoactive hormones may cause pressure diuresis. Volume depletion and hypokalemia can occur. Thus, the work-up for secondary hypertension can be confusing in the setting of accelerated hypertension.

Persistent diastolic BP higher than 130 mm Hg is often associated with acute vascular damage. Moreover, elevated BP that remains at a critical level can produce local and systemic effects that further increase BP, cause vascular damage, and eventuate in accelerated-malignant hypertension (Figure 2).

BP must be lowered but not so abruptly that cerebral blood flow is compromised. In all cases, diastolic BPs higher than 130 mm Hg should be treated. In some patients, BP should be titrated more rapidly with parenteral drugs while observing for ischemia; in others, this should be done more slowly with oral agents. Rapid normalization of BP may cause myocardial, renal, and cerebral ischemia.

In this patient, the work-up is delayed until her BP is controlled and a stable antihypertensive regimen is implemented. Her renal function and potassium levels return to normal. At follow-up 6 months later, her creatinine level is 1.4 mg/dL.

TABLE 2
Differential diagnosis of hypertensive emergency

- Acute anxiety with hyperventilation syndrome
- Acute left ventricular failure
- Brain tumor
- Cerebrovascular incident
- Collagen diseases, particularly lupus erythematosus
- Encephalitis
- Epilepsy (postictal)
- Head injury
- Hypercalcemia
- Overdose of or withdrawal from drugs such as narcotics and amphetamines
- Pheochromocytoma
- Primary aldosteronism
- Renovascular disease
- Subarachnoid hemorrhage
- Uremia

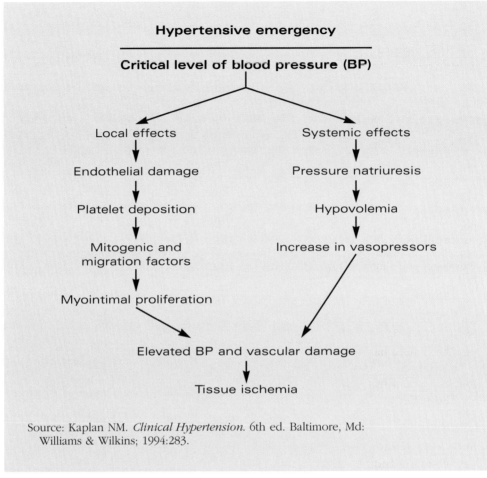

Hypertensive emergency

Critical level of blood pressure (BP)

Local effects

Endothelial damage

Platelet deposition

Mitogenic and
migration factors

Myointimal proliferation

Systemic effects

Pressure natriuresis

Hypovolemia

Increase in vasopressors

Elevated BP and vascular damage

Tissue ischemia

Source: Kaplan NM. *Clinical Hypertension.* 6th ed. Baltimore, Md:
Williams & Wilkins; 1994:283.

*Figure 2. Progression of malignant hypertension. Local and systemic effects of hypertension further
increase blood pressure and cause vascular damage and tissue ischemia.*

CLINICAL PEARLS AND PITFALLS

- Risk factors for hypertensive emergency include smoking, the use of birth control pills, and secondary causes of hypertension, such as renal artery stenosis and pheochromocytoma.
- Physical examination findings for hypertensive emergencies include retinal hemorrhage, cotton-wool spots, and papilledema.
- Hospitalization and intravenous therapy in an intensive care setting are indicated.

Additional reading

Tepel M, Zidek K. Hypertensive crisis: Pathophysiology, treatment, and handling of complications. *Kidney Int Suppl.* 1998;64:S2-S5.

Zampaglione B, Pascale C, Marchisio M, et al. Hypertensive urgencies and emergencies. Prevalence and clinical presentation. *Hypertension.* 1996;27:144-147.

Case 3. Self-assessment questions

1. Which of the following statements best characterizes this patient?
   a. The patient has acute renal failure and needs dialysis due to her altered mentation.
   b. The patient has systemic lupus erythematosus and requires corticosteroids.
   c. The patient has renovascular hypertension and requires a renal arteriogram.
   d. The patient has accelerated hypertension and requires hospitalization for treatment.
   e. The patient does not require hospitalization; she only needs sublingual nifedipine and follow-up.

2. _____ is most likely responsible for this patient's low potassium level.
   a. An aldosterone-secreting tumor
   b. Cushing's syndrome
   c. Secondary aldosteronism
   d. Chewing tobacco use
   e. Alcohol abuse

3. Among the risk factors for this patient's condition is (are) _____.
    a. low socioeconomic status
    b. secondary hypertension
    c. the use of birth control pills
    d. All of the above

4. _____ is probably responsible for the patient's mental status.
    a. Subarachnoid hemorrhage
    b. Hypertensive encephalopathy
    c. Lupus cerebritis
    d. Uremia
    e. None of the above

Answer form on page 76.

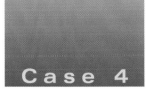

BREATHLESSNESS IN A HYPERTENSIVE AFRICAN-AMERICAN MAN

Patient presentation

A 54-year-old African-American man with a 10-year history of hypertension complains of recurring breathlessness on exertion. He denies chest heaviness, diaphoresis, or pain radiating to his throat or jaw or down his left arm. A regimen of extended-release nifedipine, 60 mg qd, and terazosin hydrochloride, 4 mg qd, reasonably controls his blood pressure (BP). He says that at home, his BP ranges 140-150/85-95 mm Hg.

He has a long-standing problem with obesity, and his weight fluctuates between 240-260 lb. His family history is remarkable for hypertension and coronary artery disease (CAD). Both his father and fraternal grandfather died in their 60s of ischemic coronary events. The patient does not smoke cigarettes. He says that he has a desk job and a sedentary lifestyle, that he rarely exercises, and that he has not had his cholesterol level measured in 10 years. Over the past year, he has gained about 10 lb. His medical history reveals an L4-L5 laminectomy for a herniated disk but is otherwise unremarkable.

Physical examination

On physical examination, the patient is 5 ft 8 in and 252 lb. His BP is 146/88 mm Hg while seated and does not vary between arms or with changes in position. His pulse is 86 beats per minute (bpm) and regular. Fundi show grade 2 hypertensive changes with some arteriolar narrowing and arteriovenous nicking. He is without carotid bruits. His lungs are clear. Cardiac examination shows a resting tachycardia with a soft systolic murmur and an S_4 gallop. His abdomen is markedly obese without organomegaly. Neurologic examination is normal. His extremities are without joint deformity or peripheral edema. He has 1+ peripheral pulses.

Laboratory evaluation

Laboratory testing reveals normal renal function and the following levels: total cholesterol, 252 mg/dL; high-density lipoprotein, 28 mg/dL; and low-density lipoprotein (LDL), 184 mg/dL. Fasting glucose level and urinalysis are normal. An electrocardiogram shows normal sinus rhythm, left axis deviation, voltage criteria for left ventricular hypertrophy, and inverted T waves in leads II, III, and aV_F. Chest film shows clear lung fields and a slightly enlarged cardiac silhouette.

Questions

What would be the optional strategy for controlling this patient's blood pressure (BP)?

To what level should his BP be reduced?

Are any additional tests required?

Discussion and management

Because this patient has a medical history of hypertension, obesity, and hyperlipidemia and a family history of CAD, he is at great risk for myocardial infarction. His recurrent breathlessness on exertion could be an anginal equivalent. Thus, a stress test with radionuclide imaging is in order to uncover any reversible ischemic defect. If such a defect is found, the patient may need coronary angiography. In turn, findings from angiography should indicate whether percutaneous transluminal coronary angioplasty or coronary artery bypass grafting is also necessary.

This patient requires both lifestyle modification and pharmacologic intervention. He needs to follow a healthier diet, with reduced intake of dietary salt, saturated fat, and calories. Pharmacologically, he will need aggressive reduction of his BP and heart rate. Although a calcium channel blocker and an α-blocker effectively control his BP, they do not reduce his heart rate, which is crucial in any antihypertensive-antianginal regimen. Reducing heart rate increases coronary artery perfusion during diastole, thus raising the threshold for an ischemic event. Conversely, accelerating the heart rate decreases coronary artery perfusion during diastole, thus lowering the threshold for such an event.

Lowering this patient's systolic BP to an optimal 130-135 mm Hg and his heart rate to 60-69 bpm should markedly reduce the ischemic burden on the left ventricle. A cardioselective or nonselective β-blocker would be best for this purpose.[1] A calcium channel blocker or a low-dose thiazide diuretic can be added, if necessary, to facilitate BP control.[2-4] Additional considerations would be drugs that inhibit the renin-angiotensin system, such as an angiotensin receptor blocker (ARB) or an angiotensin-converting enzyme (ACE) inhibitor, or an α-blocker. Both ARBs and ACE inhibitors have cardiovascular protective effects that are beneficial in patients with multiple risk factors.

This patient should also be given a hepatic hydroxymethylglutaryl coenzyme A reductase inhibitor, which will lower his LDL-cholesterol level. According to the National Cholesterol Education Program for Adult Treatment, patients with risk factors for or suspected CAD should have LDL-cholesterol levels no higher than 130 mg/dL.

CLINICAL PEARLS AND PITFALLS

- A lifestyle modification would clearly benefit in a case such as this, but because the patient has ischemic heart disease, pharmacologic efforts are also needed.
- This patient will likely require two or three drugs to control his blood pressure (BP). The β-blocker dose should be titrated upward to reduce his heart rate to 60-69 beats per minute. However, a higher dose of β-blocker—particularly a nonselective agent—could elevate his triglyceride level, which may be abnormal because of his obesity.
- Because of evidence of target organ disease, aggressive reduction in both the patient's BP and serum cholesterol levels is indicated. His systolic BP should be lowered to 130-139 mm Hg, and his low-density lipoprotein level, to under 130 mg/dL.

References
1. Yusuf S, Peto R, Lewis J, et al. Beta blockade during and after myocardial infarction: An overview of the randomized trials. *Prog Cardiovasc Dis.* 1985;27:335-371.
2. Psaty BM, Heckbert SR, Koepsell TD, et al. The risk of myocardial infarction associated with antihypertensive drug therapies. *JAMA.* 1995;274:620-625.
3. Furberg CD, Psaty BM, Meyer JV. Nifedipine. Dose-related increase in mortality in patients with coronary heart disease. *Circulation.* 1995;92:1326-1331.
4. Messerli FH. Case-control study, meta-analysis, and bouillabaisse: Putting the calcium antagonist scare into context. *Ann Intern Med.* 1995;123:888-889.

Case 4. Self-assessment questions

1. Ischemic heart disease should be treated with heart rate–lowering antihypertensive medications, such as _____.
   a. dihydropyridine calcium channel blockers
   b. cardioselective β-blockers
   c. α-blockers
   d. All of the above

2. Behavioral modification in the form of modest reductions in caloric and dietary salt intake will be helpful in this patient.
   a. True   b. False

3. An increase in heart rate shortens coronary artery perfusion time during diastole.
   a. True   b. False

4. _____ is the best way to enhance the antihypertensive activity of a β-blocker.
   a. Increasing the dose
   b. Adding low-dose hydrochlorothiazide
   c. Both a and b
   d. None of the above

Answer form on page 76.

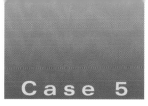

Case 5

FACIAL AND ARM NUMBNESS
IN A 64-YEAR-OLD WOMAN

Patient presentation

A 64-year-old woman presents with numbness in the left side of her face and in her left arm. About a year earlier, she came to the office and complained of headaches. At that visit, she was found to be hypertensive, with blood pressure (BP) as high as 260/136 mm Hg, and she was given an angiotensin-converting enzyme inhibitor and a calcium channel blocker. On the basis of her current symptoms, she is admitted to a local hospital.

Physical examination

On hospital admission, the patient's BP is 270/130 mm Hg. An ophthalmologist's examination discloses hypertensive hemorrhagic changes in her left eye.

Laboratory evaluation

Laboratory results show the following levels: blood urea nitrogen, 16 mg/dL; potassium, 4.4 mEq/dL; and serum creatinine, 1.0 mg/dL. The patient is given sublingual nifedipine intermittently; lisinopril, 20 mg a day; and felodipine, 5 mg once daily. Her BP is lowered to 150/70 mm Hg. A 24-hour urine collection for metanephrine catecholamines and vanillylmandelic acid is normal. An electrocardiogram shows voltage indicative of left ventricular hypertrophy.

An unenhanced computed tomography (CT) scan of the brain is normal. A CT scan of the abdomen shows an atrophic right kidney, 6 cm in length. The adrenal glands show no masses. Renal scan shows a calculated glomerular filtration rate (GFR) of 84 mL/min in the left kidney and 12 mL/min in the right kidney. Renal arteriography shows moderate arteriosclerotic changes in the aorta and iliac vessels. Nephrography shows complete occlusion of the right renal artery and mild stenosis in the proximal left renal artery.

Questions

Should any other tests be performed?

What is the diagnosis?

How should this patient be managed?

Discussion and management

Because the patient has a long history of cigarette smoking and has arteriosclerotic changes in the abdominal aorta and iliac arteries, an adenosine stress test with cardiolite is performed. The test shows normal myocardial perfusion on all tomographic sections. A right-side nephrectomy is then scheduled.

The patient tolerates the procedure well. On pathologic examination, the resected right kidney weighs 56 g. Microscopic examination shows chronic tubular interstitial nephritis and nodular hyalinizing nephrosclerosis of the renal cortex. On follow-up 2 years later, her BP remains normal, without hypertensive medication, at 120/70 mm Hg.

In a patient such as this, who is older than 50 years and who has a history of smoking and peripheral vascular disease (carotid disease), renal artery stenosis—the result of arteriosclerosis—commonly presents as accelerated malignant hypertension of short duration.[1] Diagnosis is crucial, because the condition is the most common curable cause of hypertension at any age.[2] It is also one of the few potentially reversible causes of chronic renal failure.

Although the prevalence of renovascular hypertension is not certain, it is estimated to occur in about 5% of all hypertensive patients.[2] Numerous screening techniques are available, but isotopic renography is capable of showing a markedly decreased GFR in a small right kidney. Although not performed in this case, the most sensitive screening test for renovascular hypertension is the captopril challenge test for renal blood flow. Conventional renal arteriography still provides the best anatomic imaging of the aorta, the renal artery, and the kidney.[3]

Because no image of the right kidney is visible on nephrography, renal scan shows an extremely low GFR, and a residual mass is not present, this patient is not considered a candidate for renal revascularization. Pathologic examination of the right kidney confirms the propriety of the decision for right nephrectomy.

CLINICAL PEARLS AND PITFALLS

- Patients who have atherosclerotic risk factors and who present with accelerated malignant hypertension should have aggressive work-up for renal artery stenosis, the most common curable cause of hypertension at any age.

- Although the most sensitive screening test for renovascular hypertension is the captopril renal scan, renal arteriography remains the gold standard for diagnosis.

- Surgical revascularization is the procedure of choice for cure of atherosclerotic renal artery stenosis, because the restenosis rate with angioplasty is high. Angioplasty is reserved for high-risk surgical patients and for younger patients with fibrous dysplasia.

In the Cleveland Clinic's extensive experience with surgical revascularization, hypertension is cured in 92% of patients with arteriosclerotic disease and in 90% of those with fibrous dysplasia. Percutaneous transluminal renal angioplasty is considered the procedure of choice for fibrous dysplasia. Angioplasty for arteriosclerotic renal artery stenosis is controversial, because the probability of restenosis is 30%-40%. The failure rate is particularly high with ostial stenosis.

References
1. Rimmer JM. The consequences of renal artery stenosis. *Hosp Pract.* 1994;29:29-32.
2. Pickering TG. Renovascular hypertension. In: Laragh A, Branner B, eds. *Hypertension.* New York, NY: Raven Press; 1994;1539.
3. Ram CV. Secondary hypertension: Workup and correction. *Hosp Pract.* 1994;29:137-140.

Case 5. Self-assessment questions

1. Intravenous pyelography is the most sensitive test for screening renal artery stenosis.
   a. True   b. False

2. Angioplasty is the procedure of choice for renal artery stenosis secondary to fibrous dysplasia.
   a. True   b. False

3. Renal artery stenosis is _____.
   a. the most common curable cause of hypertension
   b. estimated to occur in 5% of hypertensive patients
   c. cured surgically, when atherosclerosis is the cause
   d. All of the above

Answer form on page 76.

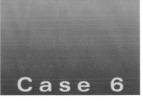

Case 6

SHORTNESS OF BREATH IN A 62-YEAR-OLD MAN

Patient presentation

A 62-year-old white man with a 20-year history of hypertension comes to the clinic and complains of shortness of breath that has worsened over the past 4 months. The patient first noticed this symptom several weeks ago while grocery shopping after a six-block walk from his home. More recently, he suffers shortness of breath with even minimal exertion, such as walking to his mailbox or taking a shower.

He began sleeping on two pillows about 2 weeks ago, because one pillow no longer sufficiently elevated his head. Shortness of breath still occasionally forces him to get up at night, however. He says that his blood pressure (BP) has not been well controlled for many years. In the past 5-6 years, he has taken numerous medications. He currently takes hydrochlorothiazide, 25 mg daily; sustained-release nifedipine, 60 mg daily; and aspirin, 325 mg daily. A chest film taken about 4 weeks ago shows an enlarged heart. An outpatient stress thallium test reveals no ischemia.

Physical examination

On physical examination his vital signs are: BP, 105/92 mm Hg; pulse, 94 beats per minute (bpm); respiratory rate, 22 breaths per minute and labored; and temperature, 97.8°F. He appears somewhat short of breath but shows no evidence of acute respiratory distress. Auscultation of the heart reveals regular heart sounds, a normal S_1 and S_2, a grade 3/6 holosystolic murmur at the apex radiating to the axilla, and an S_4 gallop. He has jugular venous distension about 8 cm above sternal angle. Examination of the lungs reveals bibasal rales halfway up the lung field, with occasional rhonchi scattered throughout both lungs. Abdominal examination shows no masses or organomegaly. The liver is not enlarged. Extremities show 1+ pitting edema over the ankles.

Laboratory evaluation

A chest film taken at this time shows evidence of bilateral pulmonary venous congestion and an enlarged heart. An electrocardiogram reveals sinus tachycardia at a rate of 106 bpm, occasional premature ventricular contractions, evidence of left ventricular and left atrial hypertrophy, and left ventricular strain pattern.

Questions

Why is this patient suffering shortness of breath and fatigue?

What are the therapeutic choices in this case?

Discussion and management

Numerous studies have shown that hypertension is an important precursor of congestive heart failure (CHF). In fact, several epidemiologic studies have shown that hypertension is the most common condition antedating CHF in the general population.

Treatment of hypertension is highly effective in reducing the incidence of CHF.[1] Recent data from the 2-year follow-up of the Framingham population, which consisted of more than 5000 patients followed up for a total of 72 422 person-years, are the best to date on the relationship between hypertension and CHF. Findings from this study show that hypertensive men and women—compared with individuals with normal BPs—have a twofold to threefold greater risk of CHF. Diabetes, left ventricular hypertrophy (LVH), and prior myocardial infarction (MI) further increase this risk. The results also show that survival following the onset of hypertensive heart failure is bleak: only 24% of patients with the disease were alive 5 years after diagnosis.

Data from the Framingham Study indicate that hypertension is the most common risk factor for CHF and that LVH is the second most important risk factor, nearly doubling the risk of heart failure in hypertensive patients overall (doubling the risk in men and tripling it in women). Diabetes is next in importance as a risk factor for CHF in hypertensive patients. Although the precise pathogenesis of heart failure in the setting of hypertension and diabetes is not fully understood, increased myocardial fibrosis may indeed play a role. The study also shows that MI has the greatest risk ratio for CHF, accounting for a nearly fivefold increase in risk for men and a sixfold increase for women.

The patient in this case has obvious clinical signs and symptoms of CHF, which is due largely to left ventricular dilatation and dysfunction, secondary to years of uncontrolled hypertension. An echocardiogram shows evidence of left ventricular enlargement, LVH, a dilated left ventricle with poor contractility, and moderate mitral valve regurgitation (Figures 1 and 2).

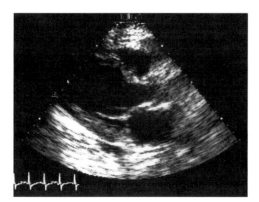

Figure 1. A two-dimensional echocardiographic image of the left ventricle in longitudinal axis. The left ventricular cavity is enlarged, and there is evidence of left ventricular hypertrophy.

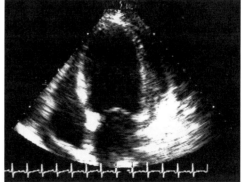

Figure 2. A two-dimensional echocardiographic image of the four chambers of the heart in the apical view. The left ventricle cavity is more than twice as large as the right ventricle, indicating significant left ventricular dilatation.

Because he has a clear clinical picture of CHF, this patient needs a significant change in his therapeutic regimen. The calcium channel blocker he is taking should be discontinued, as these drugs have been shown to increase morbidity and mortality in patients with CHF. Moreover, while hydrochlorothiazide is a good diuretic for management of hypertension, furosemide is preferable when patients are volume overloaded and congested, as is true in this case.

Ideal treatment for this patient at this stage would consist of an angiotensin receptor blocker (ARB) or an angiotensin-converting enzyme (ACE) inhibitor and furosemide. Although ACE inhibitors have long been the treatment of choice in patients with hypertension and CHF, the newer ARBs have been shown to be as effective in CHF patients.[2-4] Recent findings show that ARBs may provide better protection against the risk of sudden cardiac death,[5] are well tolerated in CHF patients,[3,4] and may regress LVH.[6]

CHF patients have many important neurohormonal abnormalities. Recent studies indicate that an increased level of plasma endothelin may be an important predictor of outcome in these patients.[2] Certain drugs have been shown to have beneficial effects on plasma endothelin levels. Results of the Fosinopril Efficacy and Safety Trial study show that treatment with the ACE inhibitor fosinopril is highly beneficial in reducing endothelin levels. This effect is subsequently correlated with significant improvement in the functional status of the patient. Evidence also exists that ACE inhibitors improve cardiac performance and normalize endothelial function in CHF patients.[2] Thus, these drugs may have important antiischemic effects, preventing further ischemic events in patients with coronary artery disease.

ARBs and ACE inhibitors are treatment of choice in patients with hypertension and CHF, because these drugs control BP, improve cardiac performance, and reduce the morbidity and mortality related to CHF. As a rule, ACE inhibitors should be initiated in small doses to avoid any risk of hypotension in patients with untreated CHF. ARBs work similarly and are not associated with intolerance. ARBs have also been shown to improve hemodynamics in CHF as well as clinical signs and symptoms of the disease.

CLINICAL PEARLS AND PITFALLS

- Hypertensive patients have a two to three times greater risk for congestive heart failure (CHF) than do normotensive patients. Treatment of hypertension has been highly effective in reducing the incidence of CHF.

- Data from the Framingham Study show hypertension to be the most common risk factor for CHF.

- Concomitant diabetes and prior myocardial infarction further increase the risk of CHF in hypertensive patients.

References

1. Deedwania PC. The progression from hypertension to heart failure. *Am J Hypertens.* 1997;10(suppl 10):280S-288S.
2. Galatius-Jensen S, Wroblewski H, Emmeluth C, et al. Plasma endothelin in congestive heart failure: Effect of the ACE inhibitor, fosinopril. *Cardiovasc Res.* 1996;32:1148-1154.
3. Nampalli V, Alhaddad IA, Denny DM, et al. Irbesartan compared with lisinopril in patients with mild to moderate heart failure [abstract]. American College of Cardiology annual meeting. March 1998. Atlanta, Ga.
4. Tonkon M, Awan N, Niazi I, et al. Irbesartan combined with conventional therapy, including angiotensin converting enzyme inhibitors, in heart failure [abstract]. American College of Cardiology annual meeting. March 1998. Atlanta, Ga.
5. Pitt B, Segal R, Martinez FA, et al. Randomised trial of losartan versus captopril in patients over 65 with heart failure. (Evaluation of Losartan in the Elderly Study, ELITE). *Lancet.* 1997;349:747-752.
6. Kahan T, Malmqvist K, Edner M, et al. Rate and extent of left ventricular hypertrophy regression: A comparison of angiotensin II blockade with irbesartan and β-blockade [abstract]. American College of Cardiology annual meeting. March 1998. Atlanta, Ga.

Case 6. Self-assessment questions

1. Myocardial infarction is the most common risk factor for congestive heart failure (CHF).

   a. True   b. False

2. The angiotensin-converting enzyme inhibitor fosinopril has been very effective in increasing plasma levels of endothelin, which may be an important predictor of outcome in CHF.

   a. True   b. False

3. Which of the following statement(s) is (are) true?

   a. Treatment of hypertension has been shown to be effective in reducing the incidence of CHF.
   b. Patients with hypertension have a twofold to threefold greater risk of CHF than do normotensive patients.
   c. In hypertensive patients with CHF, the 5-year survival rate is only 24%.
   d. All of the above

Answer form on page 76.

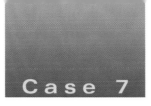

HEADACHES AND FATIGUE IN A 62-YEAR-OLD WOMAN

Patient presentation

A 62-year-old white woman with borderline hypertension complains of intermittent, retroorbital headaches and fatigue. Since her hypertension was diagnosed 10 years ago, she has taken numerous antihypertensive agents. She says that when she measures her blood pressure (BP) at home, it is usually 120-130/70-80 mm Hg. Yet, it is always much higher in the physician's office. Her previous physician told her this phenomenon was anxiety-related and prescribed the β-blocker atenolol, 50 mg qd, which she continues to take. Since she started taking atenolol, her BP is lower at home but is still not well controlled in the medical office.

Her medical history is otherwise unremarkable. Her only surgery has been a cholecystectomy. She has been modestly overweight most of her life. She denies cardiopulmonary disease, stroke, or kidney problems. She has no known allergies. Her family history is remarkable for hypertension in her mother and diabetes in her paternal grandfather. She does not smoke cigarettes or drink alcohol. She admits that she has a largely sedentary lifestyle and that she makes no effort to restrict salt or saturated fat in her diet.

Physical examination

On physical examination, the patient is 5 ft 6 in and 172 lb. Her BP is initially 148/94 mm Hg and does not change with position. Taken 10 minutes later, it is 138/90 mm Hg. Her pulse is 74 beats per minute. She is normocephalic and atraumatic. Her extraocular movements are full. Fundi show minimal hypertensive changes with some arteriolar narrowing and arteriovenous nicking. The pharynx is benign. The lungs are clear. Cardiac examination shows a regular rate and rhythm, a soft systolic murmur, and normal jugular venous pressure. The abdomen is obese and without organomegaly. Extremities are without joint deformity. There is no peripheral edema, and pulses are excellent.

Laboratory evaluation

Laboratory data show total cholesterol level, 242 mg/dL, with high-density lipoprotein, 32 mg/dL, and low-density lipoprotein, 158 mg/dL. Fasting glucose level is 22 mg/dL. Renal function and urinalysis are normal. Chest film is within normal limits. Electrocardiogram shows voltage criteria for left ventricular hypertrophy (LVH).

Questions

Is this patient a candidate for pharmacotherapy?

Would any additional tests help determine whether antihypertensive therapy is necessary?

Which blood pressure readings—those taken at home or in the office—should be used to determine treatment?

Discussion and management

White coat hypertension, as illustrated in the patient in this case, is a common problem in clinical practice. She is currently taking a medication that is causing adverse effects. The question is, does she need medication at all? Unfortunately, there is no correct answer.

BP is dynamic, varying diurnally. Readings are higher during the day, particularly in the morning, than they are at night. Thus, it is not all that surprising when a BP reading taken at home in the evening varies considerably from one taken in the medical office in the morning. Consequently, BP readings at home should be recorded in the morning—and before any medication is taken. Readings in the physician's office should be similarly timed.

It may seem logical that BP readings taken at home, while the patient is relaxed, are lower than those taken in the physician's office, which is a more stressful environment. Nevertheless, physicians have four decades of experience treating hypertension based on office determinations of BP. If office-based readings are repeatedly elevated, lowering both systolic and diastolic BP has been shown to reduce morbidity and mortality.

No data exist on treating hypertension on the basis of home readings. Nor is there any information on outcomes using data obtained from 24-hour ambulatory monitoring. For these reasons, an appropriate and conservative approach is to base pharmacotherapy decisions on repeated office measurements. Physicians must also be sensitive to the fact that patients taking medication for hypertension diagnosed with office BP readings may have episodes of symptomatic hypotension at home. If so, it is time to reevaluate the antihypertensive strategy and consider 24-hour ambulatory BP monitoring.

Clinical studies suggest that not all white coat hypertensive patients are the same. Some have cardiovascular risk clustering factors. Others do not. In certain patients, white coat hypertension could indicate the subsequent risks of sustained hypertension and target organ damage. Clinical trials are currently underway to analyze these differences and their impact on treatment.

Meanwhile, medical office staff should measure a patient's BP at the same time of day that the patient measures it at home. The BP measuring equipment that the patient uses at home should provide similar readings to the mercury sphygmomanometer used in the physician's office. For this reason, any BP monitoring device used in a patient's home should be tested in the physician's office. Vast discrepancies in BP should be checked with 24-hour ambulatory BP monitoring. The persistence of symptomatic hypertension, despite aggressive treatment based on office determinations, also indicates ambulatory BP monitoring.

This patient's family history of hypertension, mild dyslipidemia, early evidence of LVH, and obesity encourage more aggressive strategies to control her BP. Because she is postmenopausal, she may also be a candidate for estrogen replacement therapy. In a patient such as this, who has coexisting cardiovascular risk factors, optimal BP should be 130/85 mm Hg or lower.

Since she appears to be having symptoms related to the β-blockers, an alternative form of pharmacotherapy should be chosen. Appropriate therapy would consist of any of a number of different medications, including an angiotensin receptor blocker, an angiotensin-converting enzyme inhibitor, a calcium channel blocker, or any form of pharmacotherapy that effectively controls BP yet causes minimal adverse effects. She should also be encouraged to exercise, lose weight, and modestly reduce her dietary salt intake.

CLINICAL PEARLS AND PITFALLS

- The patient should be informed that blood pressures (BP) measured at home and in the medical office may differ widely and that measuring BP at the same time of day in both environments helps to reduce these differences.
- BP measurements taken with a home monitoring device should be compared with those taken with the mercury sphygmomanometer used in the physician's office.
- Because this patient has at least two cardiovascular risk factors, her optimal BP should be lower than 130/85 mm Hg.
- Optimal treatment for this patient is both nonpharmacologic and pharmacologic. A pharmacologic agent should be selected for its efficacy as well as its tolerability.

Additional reading

Mancia G, Bertinieri G, Grassi G, et al. Effects of blood pressure measurement by the doctor on patient's blood pressure and heart rate. *Lancet*. 1983;2:695-698.

Meredith PA, Perloff D, Mancia G, et al. Blood pressure variability and its implications for antihypertensive therapy. *Blood Press*. 1995;4:5-11.

Muller JE, Stone PH, Turi ZG, et al. Circadian variation in the frequency of onset of acute myocardial infarction. *N Engl J Med*. 1985;313:1315-1322.

Pickering TG, James GD, Boddie C, et al. How common is white coat hypertension? *JAMA*. 1988;259:225-228.

Case 7. Self-assessment questions

1. White coat hypertension results from excess activity of the sympathetic nervous system.
   a. True   b. False

2. Optimal treatment for white coat hypertension is a β-blocker.
   a. True   b. False

3. White coat hypertension may be related to the time of day when blood pressure (BP) is measured. Diurnal variation in BP is evidenced by higher BPs during the day and lower BPs at night.
   a. True   b. False

4. Decades of experience in treating hypertension show that reducing BP on the basis of office measurements correlates with reduced morbidity and mortality.
   a. True   b. False

Answer form on page 76.

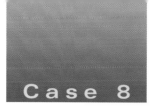

Case 8

CHEST PAIN IN A 46-YEAR-OLD AFRICAN-AMERICAN MAN

Patient presentation

A 46-year-old African-American man with long-standing hypertension comes to the office and describes substernal chest pain during sexual intercourse and after climbing two flights of stairs. He says his symptoms began about a month ago. He adds that he feels relief within 5 minutes of stopping the provoking activity.

He is currently taking a long-acting dihydropyridine calcium antagonist to control his blood pressure (BP). He does not take his medication consistently, however, because of the associated peripheral edema. His previous physician switched his medications many times over the years because of side effects. The patient says that he has never taken a combination of drugs, only one drug at a time. With him, he has a record of his BP readings—most higher than 160/98 mm Hg—taken over 2 years of office visits.

He does not smoke cigarettes. Nor does he have diabetes or a lipid disorder. He admits that he does exercise. He is a successful businessman, and his work is stressful. He drinks three gin and tonics each evening. He denies the use of illicit drugs. His family history is strongly positive for cardiovascular disease and hypertension. His mother died at 54 years of age, and his father, at 47 years, of a cerebrovascular accident. His older brother had a myocardial infarction (MI) at the age of 50 years. All family members have hypertension.

Physical examination

The patient's BP is 184/104 mm Hg and does not vary between arms. Pulse is 98 beats per minute. Examination of the fundi shows arteriolar narrowing and arteriovenous crossing changes without hemorrhages or exudates. There is no jugular venous distention, carotid bruits, or thyromegaly. There are no crackles or wheezes. An S_4 gallop and sustained left ventricular impulse are present. Abdominal examination is unremarkable. All pulses in the upper and lower extremities are equal.

Laboratory findings

A complete blood count and sequential multiple analyses are normal. An electrocardiogram (ECG) shows increased voltage and a strain pattern (Figure 1). An echocardiogram shows left ventricular hypertrophy (LVH), good left ventricular performance, and no wall motion abnormalities. An exercise stress test shows 2-mm ST depression beyond baseline changes. Cardiac catheterization shows mostly normal coronary arteries, with luminal irregularities.

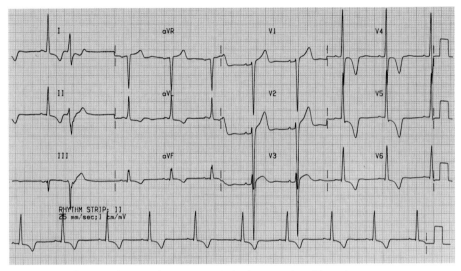

Figure 1. An electrocardiogram showing ventricular hypertrophy with strain.

Questions

Should any additional tests be performed?

How should this patient be managed?

Discussion and management

This case illustrates several points. MI may occur in a hypertensive patient as a result of large vessel coronary artery disease (CAD), acute aortic dissection, small vessel disease, medial vessel hypertrophy, or an inadequate coronary blood flow for the amount of myocardium perfused (coronary flow reserve abnormality). Physicians must ask about precipitating causes (including drugs such as cocaine, phenylpropanolamine, and ergot preparations), carefully examine for dissection and clues of atherosclerosis (carotid, femoral, and abdominal bruits), and exclude large vessel disease (because of the potential for revascularization).

In this case, the ECG shows LVH with nonspecific ST-T wave changes. This finding increases the risk of CAD and excludes the need for a routine exercise stress test. With only LVH, the overall accuracy of a Bruce treadmill is 42% in hypertensive patients. Exercise radionuclide ventriculography is associated with a false-positive rate of 75% and an overall accuracy of 49%. Exercise thallium is associated with a false-positive rate of 36% and an overall accuracy of 70%. It is a reasonable test of exclusion for epicardial CAD. Although exercise echocardiography provides more data, it is not advantageous in all patients, since the acoustic window for judging wall motion abnormalities may not be optimal. Contrast and tissue perfusion may broaden the usefulness of stress echocardiography.

This patient may need multiple drugs, such as an angiotensin receptor blocker (ARB) with hydrochlorothiazide (HCTZ) or an angiotensin-converting enzyme (ACE) inhibitor with HCTZ, to lower his BP. An ARB combination with HCTZ is a good choice for him. Although many African Americans have low-renin hypertension and do not respond to ACE inhibition, preliminary data suggest that ARBs with diuretics are effective in this patient population.

Generally, patients should be counseled to limit their ethanol intake to 1 oz of equivalent alcohol. Alcohol elevates BP acutely and chronically. Heavy alcohol intake is associated with a higher rate of intracerebral hemorrhage, but decreasing his overall ethanol intake could reduce the number.

CLINICAL PEARLS AND PITFALLS

- Myocardial ischemia may develop in hypertensive patients due to aortic dissection, small vessel disease, coronary flow reserve abnormality, or—most commonly—coronary artery disease.
- Routine exercise stress testing (EST) has lower specificity than EST-thallium, sestamibi, or echocardiography in hypertensive patients.

Additional reading

Houghton JL, Prisant LM, Carr AA, et al. Relationship of left ventricular mass to impairment of coronary vasodilator reserve in hypertensive heart disease. *Am Heart J.* 1991;121:1107-1112.

Prisant LM, Frank MJ, Carr AA, et al. How can we diagnose coronary heart disease in hypertensive patients? *Hypertension.* 1987;10:467-472.

Case 8. Self-assessment questions

1. The best explanation for this patient's chest pain is _____.
   a. coronary artery spasm
   b. a significant lesion, which was missed on the coronary arteriogram
   c. an inadequate coronary flow reserve
   d. a noncardiac cause
   e. an adverse drug reaction

2. In patients with hypertension with or without left ventricular hypertrophy, the negative predictive value of a test to assess for epicardial coronary artery disease is highest with _____.
   a. a standard Bruce exercise stress test
   b. exercise nuclear ventriculography
   c. thallium stress test
   d. dobutamine stress echocardiography

3. Hypertensive patients may experience myocardial ischemia on the basis of _____.
   a. atherosclerotic narrowing of the epicardial coronary arteries
   b. impaired coronary flow reserve
   c. small vessel (intramural) coronary disease
   d. dissection of the aorta
   e. All of the above

4. _____ elevate(s) blood pressure and cause(s) coronary vasoconstriction or spasm.
   a. Cocaine
   b. Phenylpropanolamine (in weight-reducing preparations and cold remedies)
   c. Phenylephrine (in nose drops)
   d. Ergot preparations (for migraine)
   e. All of the above

Answer form on page 76.

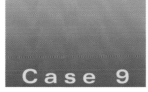

Case 9

EXERTIONAL CHEST PAIN
IN A 54-YEAR-OLD HYPERTENSIVE MAN

Patient presentation

A 54-year-old Hispanic man has had exertional chest pain for the past 2 months.
He says that he first noticed the pain in the left side of his chest while he was lifting
some heavy objects at work. The pain lasted only about 5 minutes and was relieved
with rest. Since then, he has had two or three additional episodes, usually when
walking fast or lifting something heavy. In these instances, the chest pain again
lasted only a few minutes and was relieved spontaneously.

The patient has a 12-year history of diabetes mellitus and a 7-year history of
hypertension. For the last 2 years, he has taken insulin, 15 units in the morning,
to control his blood sugar level. He also follows a diabetic diet. He has a strong
family history of diabetes. His mother, aunt, and older brother have the disease and
take insulin. When the patient's hypertension was diagnosed 7 years ago, he began
taking hydrochlorothiazide, 25 mg daily, and atenolol, 50 mg daily, which he still
takes. Over the years, these medications have controlled his blood pressure (BP)
reasonably well. He claims that it is usually 140/90 mm Hg.

Physical examination

Physical examination reveals a well-built and well-nourished man, who appears his
age. He is 5 ft 6 in and 200 lb. Vital signs are: BP, 140/85 mm Hg; pulse, 72 beats per
minute (bpm); respiratory rate, 16 breaths per minute; and temperature, 98.4°F. Cardiac
examination reveals a regular rhythm, with no murmur or gallops. Examination of the
lungs reveals clear breath sounds. His abdomen has no masses or organomegaly.
Bowel sounds are present. His extremities show no edema, but the dorsalis pedis
pulse on the left foot is feeble. Neurologic examination shows no evidence of
peripheral neuropathy or gross focal defects.

Laboratory evaluation

An electrocardiogram (ECG) reveals normal sinus rhythm at a rate of 76 bpm, left
atrial enlargement, and borderline voltage criteria for left ventricular hypertrophy
(LVH). There is no evidence of ST-T wave changes. Fasting glucose level is 130
mg/dL, and serum creatinine level is 1.6 mg/dL. Hemoglobin A_{1C} is 7.2%. Urinalysis
reveals microalbuminuria. A chest film is unremarkable. There is no evidence of
cardiomegaly or pulmonary congestion.

Questions

What diagnostic test should be performed to evaluate the patient's chest pain?

What is the significance of microalbuminuria on urinalysis in this patient?

Should the patient's treatment regimen be changed?

Discussion and management

Hypertension and diabetes commonly coexist. A recent survey shows that of approximately 8 million Americans who have diabetes, nearly 3 million—about 40%—also have hypertension, and patients with both disorders are at increased risk for coronary artery disease (CAD). The two disorders act synergistically to accelerate the overall atherosclerotic process, thereby increasing the risk of myocardial infarction. The coexistence of diabetes and hypertension also increases the risk of cardiomyopathy.

Numerous mechanisms for cardiomyopathy have been suggested in patients with concomitant hypertension and diabetes. The most accepted theories relate to an increased risk of LVH and left ventricular wall thickness and to an increased amount of dense interstitial connective tissue throughout the myocardium, as evidenced in autopsy specimens. Echocardiographic studies have also shown increased left ventricular mass in hypertensive diabetic patients. Compared with hypertensive patients without diabetes, hypertensive patients with diabetes are at significantly greater risk for diastolic dysfunction. Patients with both disorders are also at significantly increased risk for nephropathy, retinopathy, cardiovascular and cerebral vascular events, and peripheral vascular disease.

This patient's 2-month history of exertional chest pain is highly suggestive of underlying CAD. Because his baseline 12-lead ECG is normal, the ideal test for him now is an exercise treadmill, with either an echocardiogram or nuclear imaging, to detect exertional myocardial ischemia. The treadmill test is performed and reveals a 1.5-mm ST-T segment depression in inferior leads, with inferior wall ischemia on thallium images. These findings indicate the presence of exercise-induced myocardial ischemia. The patient is given sublingual nitroglycerin, 0.4 mg (1/150 grain), as needed for chest pain, and his once-daily dose of the β blocker atenolol is increased from 50 to 75 mg.

Recent studies indicate that microalbuminuria—which this patient has—in the setting of diabetes and hypertension is associated with significantly increased risk of CAD. The patient's exercise test confirms the presence of CAD. He should be carefully evaluated for all coexisting coronary risk factors. Effective control of BP and glucose metabolism in this patient can reduce his risk of cardiovascular complications. Although many drugs that are effective in hypertensive patients have been tried in diabetic patients, some routinely used hypertensive agents may not be suitable. Diuretics, particularly thiazide diuretics, have been shown to decrease insulin sensitivity, impair glucose tolerance, and produce hyperglycemia. Moreover, certain calcium channel blockers, such as the dihydropyridines, can adversely affect glucose metabolism.

Changing his therapeutic regimen should be considered. He is presently taking hydrochlorothiazide, a diuretic, which as previously noted, is not a good choice for a diabetic patient. An angiotensin-converting enzyme (ACE) inhibitor would be a valuable addition to his therapeutic armamentarium. ACE inhibitors are reasonably safe, well tolerated, and highly effective in patients with hypertension and diabetes. These drugs have a distinct advantage over others in these patients, because they are highly effective in reducing BP without adversely affecting blood glucose metabolism.

ACE inhibitors can also blunt the rise in microalbuminuria, increase insulin sensitivity, and slow the progression of diabetic nephropathy. Compared with placebo, captopril has been shown to reduce the rate of doubling of serum creatinine levels, the need for dialysis and renal transplantation, and the risk of death.[1,2] Although ACE inhibitors can deteriorate renal function, especially in patients with preexisting renal disease, drugs such as fosinopril may be safer than others due to their dual route (hepatobiliary and renal) of elimination.[3] Although angiotensin receptor blockers (ARBs) are well tolerated, the role of ARBs has not yet been defined in this population.

The National High Blood Pressure Education Program Working Group recently issued a report on the treatment of hypertension in diabetic patients.[4] This report supports the facts that the concurrence of these two diseases increases morbidity and mortality and that ACE inhibitors, and possibly ARBs, provide benefits in such settings.

CLINICAL PEARLS AND PITFALLS

- Patients with concomitant hypertension and diabetes are at increased risk for nephropathy; retinopathy; and cardiovascular, cerebrovascular, and peripheral vascular disorders.

- Treatment of hypertension with angiotensin-converting enzyme (ACE) inhibitors slows the progression of diabetic nephropathy.

- Effective control of blood pressure and glucose metabolism can reduce the risk of cardiovascular complications in hypertensive diabetic patients. ACE inhibitors are now considered first-line therapy for these patients.

References

1. Rodby RA, Rohde R, Evans J, et al. The study of the effect of intensity of blood pressure management on the progression of type 1 diabetic nephropathy: Study design and baseline patient characteristics. The Collaborative Study Group. *J Am Soc Nephrol.* 1995;5:1775-1781.
2. Breyer JA, Bain RP, Evans JK, et al. Predictors of the progression of renal insufficiency in patients with insulin-dependent diabetes and overt diabetic nephropathy. The Collaborative Study Group. *Kidney Int.* 1996;50:1651-1658.
3. Mancia G, Giannattasio C, Grassi G. Treatment of heart failure with fosinopril: An angiotensin converting enzyme inhibitor with a dual and compensatory route of excretion. *Am J Hypertens.* 1997;10(suppl 10):236S-241S.
4. National High Blood Pressure Education Program Working Group. 1995 update of the working group reports on chronic renal failure and renovascular hypertension. *Arch Intern Med.* 1996;156:1938-1947.

Case 9. Self-assessment questions

1. Patients with concomitant hypertension and diabetes are at markedly increased risk for diabetic nephropathy.
   a. True   b. False

2. Patients with concomitant hypertension and diabetes are at significantly greater risk for diastolic dysfunction than are hypertensive patients without diabetes.
   a. True   b. False

3. Which of the following statements about drugs used to treat hypertension in diabetic patients is *not* true?
   a. Angiotensin-converting enzyme (ACE) inhibitors slow the progression of diabetic nephropathy.
   b. Thiazide diuretics impair glucose metabolism.
   c. Certain calcium channel blockers can have an adverse impact on glucose metabolism.
   d. ACE inhibitors decrease insulin sensitivity.

Answer form on page 76.

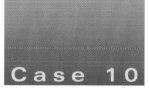

Case 10

NONCOMPLIANCE IN A HYPERTENSIVE PATIENT

Patient presentation

A 36-year-old African-American man with uncontrolled hypertension comes to the office. In the 12 years since his diagnosis, his high blood pressure (BP) has been resistant to nearly all medications, including calcium channel blockers, angiotensin-converting enzyme (ACE) inhibitors, β-blockers, and α-blockers. Moreover, he has experienced troubling side effects: Calcium channel blockers made his ankles swell. ACE inhibitors gave him a cough. β- and α-blockers made him tired, reduced his libido, and caused episodes of impotence. And diuretics gave him cramps.

The patient is an accountant. He does not smoke cigarettes or drink alcohol. He exercises daily and plays competitive basketball on weekends. His weight remains stable, and he has been physically fit his entire life. He has tried to reduce his salt intake and to avoid saturated fat, but his busy lifestyle and frequent need to entertain clients and friends have made this difficult.

His medical history is largely unremarkable. Despite his prolonged hypertension, he has had no medical problems other than occasional headaches. His family history is strong for hypertension on both sides. Several relatives had coronary artery disease, and two grandparents died in their 60s of stroke.

Physical examination

The patient appears healthy. He is 6 ft 0 in and 185 lb. His BP is 188/112 mm Hg while seated and does not change with position. His pulse is 62 beats per minute and regular. Funduscopy shows arteriolar narrowing and arteriovenous nicking. His pharynx is benign. He has 2+ carotid pulses. His chest is clear. His cardiac examination shows an S_4 gallop and a palpable, laterally displaced point of maximal intensity. Abdominal examination is benign. He is without scars, masses, tenderness, or organomegaly. Neurologic examination shows no focal deficits or pathologic reflexes. Peripheral pulses in the extremities are excellent, and there is no joint deformity or edema.

Laboratory evaluation

Laboratory tests reveal the following levels: blood urea nitrogen, 19 mg/dL; creatinine, 1.5 mg/dL; total cholesterol, 202 mg/dL; high-density lipoprotein, 48 mg/dL; and low-density lipoprotein, 122 mg/dL. He has a normal fasting glucose. Urinalysis shows a specific gravity of 1.020; 1+ protein; 0-2 white cells per high-power field, 0-2 red cells, and no bacteria. Electrocardiogram shows voltage consistent for left ventricular hypertrophy and nonspecific ST-T wave changes.

Questions

What would be the optimal strategy for controlling this young man's blood pressure?

Is his hypertension primary or secondary?

How can compliance be improved in a patient who has had adverse effects with most antihypertensive medications?

Discussion and management

This young man has significant hypertensive disease that has already affected two major target organs—the heart and kidneys. Although it is likely that he has familial essential hypertension, the mild increase in his creatinine level and 1+ dipstick for protein could indicate early kidney disease. Thus, additional evaluation should include a 24-hour urine collection, a renal sonogram, and possibly a kidney biopsy.

Another major problem in this case is how to manage a young and healthy patient who has experienced adverse events with antihypertensive medications. The physician should carefully review the agents and doses given and the side effects that ensued. The problem may have been that the doses were too high or that the course of medication was too short to establish its efficacy and tolerability.

The physician should also assess the patient's knowledge about the importance of BP control and about target organ damage. Moreover, the need for good doctor-patient dialogue should be emphasized to facilitate an appropriate choice of therapy. Noncompliance often results from a hypertensive patient's lack of understanding of the need to treat an asymptomatic disease. In many other cases, patients are unwilling to tell their physician that a medication is causing them problems. Rather than complain about a drug's adverse events, they simply stop taking it. Consequently, their hypertension remains uncontrolled. The physician may see this as the medication's lack of efficacy. Clearly, educating patients about the necessity of BP control is pivotal in treatment success.

This patient will probably require multiple drugs to control his BP. Because of his markedly elevated diastolic and systolic pressures and his early evidence of renal dysfunction, a rational strategy would consist of two or more agents given in low doses over 6-12 weeks. The combination of a thiazide diuretic and a drug that inhibits the renin-angiotensin (RA) system with or without a calcium channel blocker would be ideal.

This patient is an ideal candidate for combination therapy with an angiotensin receptor blocker (ARB) and hydrochlorothiazide (HCTZ). Data show that ARBs reverse progression of LVH and when used in combination with HCTZ, markedly reduce BP. They are cardioprotective and provide end organ protection. Because ARBs have a side effect profile similar to that of placebo, they are well-suited to this patient, who has had problems with adverse effects from other medications.

Diuretic support may be necessary due to the patient's mild renal insufficiency. Thiazide diuretics have been shown to work well in African-American hypertensive patients and with drugs that block the RA system. Adding a calcium channel blocker may augment the antihypertensive capabilities of the other two drugs. Much as an ACE inhibitor does, an ARB may reduce the risk of leg edema that is associated with calcium channel blockers.

This patient should continue attempts to maintain ideal body weight, to exercise regularly, and to avoid processed foods, which contain considerable amounts of salt and can antagonize the antihypertensive properties of his medications. He should be encouraged to call his physician with any problems. He might also be instructed on how to monitor his BP at home, so that he will know when his clinical condition has improved.

CLINICAL PEARLS AND PITFALLS

- Patients should have an interest in their clinical care. They should be well educated about the problems associated with uncontrolled hypertension and the need for blood pressure (BP) control.

- Noncompliance is often related to adverse events. In patients who have had problems with side effects, lower doses of two or more drugs may be ideal. The patient in this case has evidence of kidney disease, perhaps because of his high BP or underlying disease. This condition should be carefully evaluated and treated, if necessary.

Additional reading

Epstein M, Bakris G. Newer approaches to antihypertensive therapy. Use of fixed-dose combination therapy. *Arch Intern Med.* 1996;156:1969-1978.

Neutel JM, Black HR, Weber MA. Combination therapy with diuretics: An evolution of understanding. *Am J Med.* 1996;101:61S-70S.

Weir MR, Prisant LM, Papademetriou V, et al. Antihypertensive therapy and quality of life. Influence of blood pressure reduction, adverse events, and prior antihypertensive therapy. *Am J Hypertens.* 1996;9:854-859.

Case 10: Self-assessment questions

1. Evaluation of a hypertensive patient with a mildly increased serum creatinine level and dipstick positive proteinuria should include a 24-hour creatinine clearance and protein assessment, a renal sonogram, and a possible kidney biopsy.
   a. True   b. False

2. Thiazide diuretics have been shown to work well in African-American hypertensive patients and with drugs that block the renin-angiotensin system.
   a. True   b. False

3. Lower doses of two or more drugs may be ideal in patients who are often symptomatic with single drugs titrated to higher doses.
   a. True   b. False

Answer form on page 76.

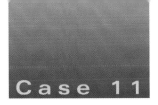

DYSPNEA IN A 57-YEAR-OLD WHITE MAN

Patient presentation

A 57-year-old white man with a 15-year history of hypertension comes to the office and says that for the past 3 weeks, he has had difficulty breathing after climbing a flight of stairs. He denies orthopnea, paroxysmal nocturnal dyspnea, cough, wheezes, fever, or chills. He has no history of chest pain, palpitations, syncope, claudication, myocardial infarction (MI), or stroke. He stopped smoking cigarettes 25 years earlier. He does not know his cholesterol level. He has been unable to afford his antihypertensive medications for several months.

Physical examination

On physical examination, the patient's vital signs are: blood pressure (BP), 162/108 mm Hg; pulse, 98 beats per minute; respiration, 14 breaths per minute. He is 5 ft 10 in and 220 lb. There is no icterus. Funduscopic examination shows arteriovenous crossing changes, but there are no hemorrhages, exudates, or papilledema. There is no jugular venous distention at 30°, and there are no carotid bruits. The thyroid gland is unremarkable.

Auscultation of the lungs does not reveal any rales or wheezes. The left ventricular apical impulse is displaced outside the midclavicular line, enlarged in diameter, and sustained. Cardiac rhythm is regular. The S_1 is within normal limits, and the S_2 is split physiologically. There is a loud S_4 but no S_3 gallop. A grade 2/6 systolic ejection murmur can be heard at the left sternal border and apex. Abdominal examination reveals no enlargement of the liver or spleen. Bowel sounds are normoactive. No abdominal or femoral bruits are detected. Peripheral pulses are 2+ and equal in the upper and lower extremities, and there is no clubbing, cyanosis, or edema.

Laboratory examination

Laboratory tests show the following levels: creatinine, 1.6 mg/dL; fasting cholesterol, 268 mg/dL; triglycerides, 200 mg/dL; glucose, 145 mg/dL. Sequential multiple analysis is otherwise normal, as is the complete blood count. Urinalysis shows 2+ proteinuria. An electrocardiogram (ECG) is also performed.

Questions

What criteria are most reliable in diagnosing left ventricular hypertrophy?

Should any additional tests be performed?

Discussion and management

Left ventricular hypertrophy (LVH) is the consequence of uncontrolled hypertension; it is also the most significant cardiovascular risk factor. It is an independent risk factor for MI, stroke, sudden death, and congestive heart failure. The Sixth Report of the Joint National Committee (JNC VI) on Prevention, Detection, Evaluation, and Treatment of High Blood Pressure considers the diagnosis of LVH important in risk stratification and treatment.[1]

In identifying LVH, a boot-shaped heart on a chest film is neither a sensitive nor specific marker. Rather, the presence of an enlarged (>3 cm), sustained left ventricular impulse on physical examination suggests the diagnosis. Although there are numerous ECG criteria for LVH, the gender-specific Cornell criteria have greater sensitivity (30%) without sacrificing specificity (80%) (Table 1). In the Framingham Study, the repolarization abnormality, or strain pattern, in the lateral precordial leads is associated with death within 5 years in 33% of men and 21% of women. Because ECG manifestations of LVH do not occur early, they are not sensitive.

While magnetic resonance imaging is the most sensitive and accurate method for detecting LVH, it is not practical in most patients. An echocardiogram is useful if the image and measurements are acquired with meticulous attention. This method not only relays left atrial size and left ventricular wall thickness and chamber dimensions, it also provides data on left ventricular performance and evidence of previous MI.

Although ECGs and echocardiograms provide complementary information, an echocardiogram is not necessary in the routine initial work-up of a hypertensive patient. In this patient, however, it may be useful in evaluating his dyspnea. If the ejection fraction is normal, any therapy that lowers BP will result in decreased left end-diastolic pressure and left atrial pressure. If the ejection fraction is low, antihypertensive drugs that are myocardial depressants would have to be used cautiously.

TABLE 1
Cornell criteria for left ventricular hypertrophy

- $RaV_L + SV_3$ = total voltage

- Abnormal total voltage >2.8 mV in men and >2.0 mV in women

An echocardiogram is ordered for this patient and shows normal left ventricular function (ejection fraction of 74%) and a moderate increase in wall thickness. The patient is educated about the target organ damage (LVH and renal insufficiency) already present and his coexisting risk factors. He is also informed that intensive dietary therapy with weight loss should help his glucose intolerance, lipid disorder, and hypertension.

According to the JNC VI, pharmacologic therapy is indicated for high normal BP (130-139/85-80 mm Hg) in the presence of target organ damage or clinical cardiovascular disease. Data show that angiotensin receptor blockers (ARBs) and angiotensin-converting enzyme (ACE) inhibitors reverse the progression of LVH. This patient began concentrated treatment with an ARB. At follow-up, drug therapy and weight loss improved his dyspnea and overall cardiovascular profile.

CLINICAL PEARLS AND PITFALLS

- Left ventricular hypertrophy (LVH) secondary to hypertension is the most potent of all cardiovascular risk factors. It is an independent risk factor for congestive heart failure, myocardial infarction, stroke, and sudden death.

- Cornell criteria are the most sensitive electrocardiographic markers for diagnosing LVH.

- Although magnetic resonance imaging is the most sensitive test for diagnosing LVH, it is costly. Consequently, echocardiography is the technique most widely used to identify LVH.

Reference

1. The Sixth Report of the Joint National Committee on Prevention, Detection, Evaluation, and Treatment of High Blood Pressure. Bethesda, Md: National Institutes of Health, NHLBI. 1997. NIH 98-4080.

Additional reading

Crow RS, Hannan P, Grandits G, et al. Is the echocardiogram an appropriate ECG validity standard for the detection and change in left ventricular size? *J Electrocardiol.* 1996; 29(suppl):248-255.

Okin PM, Roman MJ, Devereux, RB, et al. Electrographic identification of increased left ventricular mass by simple voltage-duration products. *J Am Coll Cardiol.* 1995;25:417-423.

Case 11. Self-assessment questions

1. This hypertensive patient's most potent risk factor is _____.
   a. a history of tobacco use
   b. glucose intolerance
   c. a lipid disorder
   d. left ventricular hypertrophy (LVH)
   e. proteinuria

2. The electrocardiogram (ECG) suggests LVH. What component of the ECG is associated with the greatest risk?
   a. Increased voltage
   b. Left axis deviation
   c. Left atrial enlargement
   d. Increased ventricular activation time
   e. Repolarization abnormality

3. _____ is the most sensitive test for detecting LVH.
   a. Magnetic resonance imaging
   b. Echocardiogram
   c. ECG
   d. Physical examination
   e. Chest film

4. _____ criteria are the most sensitive electrocardiographic markers for detecting LVH.
   a. Sokolow-Lyons
   b. Romhilt-Estes
   c. Cornell
   d. Minnesota
   e. Oslo

Answer form on page 76.

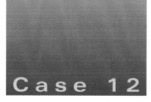

Case 12

HEADACHES, CHEST PAIN, AND FATIGUE IN A 52-YEAR-OLD MAN

Patient presentation

A 52-year-old man comes to the office and describes occipital headaches and atypical chest pain. His medical records show a recent onset of hypertension, which is associated with multiple complaints. The most distressing is morning fatigue, even after 7-8 hours of sleep. He is an avid outdoorsman and was hunting in a tick-infested area within the past month.

Physical examination

Blood pressure (BP) is 192/110 mm Hg. Funduscopic examination is normal. The lungs are clear. Cardiovascular examination shows a normal point of maximal intensity and normal heart sounds. The liver and spleen are not palpable. The extremities show no joint deformities and no edema.

Laboratory evaluation

An initial 12-lead electrocardiogram is normal. Laboratory results show normal levels of fasting blood sugar, blood urea nitrogen, serum creatinine, serum potassium, and hemoglobin. His erythrocyte sedimentation rate is also normal. Immunologic tests are negative for Lyme disease. Dual isotope imaging with thallium-201 and technetium-99m-sestamibi shows normal myocardial perfusion During exercise, the patient's maximal BP is 208/73 mm Hg.

Questions

What is the diagnosis?

Are any additional tests needed to confirm the diagnosis?

Discussion and management

Initial therapy is with lisinopril, 10 mg per day, but the patient's BP response is only modest. About 2 weeks later, the dose is increased to 20 mg per day, but his BP remains at 180/110 mm Hg. Atenolol, 50 mg per day, is then added to the regimen. After 2 additional weeks, his BP is still elevated at 172/102 mm Hg, and he continues to complain of headaches and fatigue. The lisinopril is stopped, and therapy with amlodipine, 5 mg per day, is initiated. Because the patient suffers a generalized rash 48 hours after the first dose of amlodipine, the medication is discontinued. A short course of prednisone is then administered. This is followed by therapy with extended-release verapamil hydrochloride, 240 mg daily.

In a discussion with the patient's wife, she mentions that her husband has snored loudly for years. On the basis of this information, he is sent to the sleep laboratory, where a polysomnographic study shows moderate obstructive sleep apnea (OSA). Continuous positive airway pressure (CPAP) is administered, and his condition improves. His BP prior to sleeping is 160/90 mm Hg and postsleep, decreases to 158/84 mm Hg. Some 2 months later, on follow-up of the use of nasal CPAP, BP is reduced to 138/80 mm Hg. No change is made in the patient's atenolol or verapamil.

Sleep apnea is defined as respiratory cessation for at least 10 seconds per hour for five or more periods during sleep. In its most common form—OSA—breathing efforts continue, but upper airway obstruction blocks air movement.[1] In medical outpatient clinics, the incidence of OSA in hypertensive patients ranges from 26%-48%. In the general population, about 4% of adult men and 2% of adult women have symptomatic OSA.[2] An overnight sleep study, which continuously records respiration, electroencephalographic and electrocardiographic data, and oxygen saturation, must confirm the diagnosis.

The apnea-induced increase in arterial BP can be substantial (20-40 mm Hg in systolic BP and to a lesser degree in diastolic BP). Obesity almost always accompanies OSA and leads to upper airway narrowing, glottic obstruction, and potential pulmonary failure. It is closely correlated to a higher prevalence of hypertension.

Weight loss and nasal CPAP may provide relief to massively obese patients. A dose of clonidine, 0.2 mg, administered orally at bedtime totally suppresses rapid eye movement sleep, which is associated with hypertonia in the upper airway.[3] Sleep also greatly reduces the overall ventilatory response to hypoxia and other respiratory reflexes. Patients with severe sleep apnea may require corrective surgery, which may produce a dramatic relief in hypertension.

CLINICAL PEARLS AND PITFALLS

- Sleep apnea is defined as respiratory cessation for at least 10 seconds per hour for five or more periods during sleep.

- Apnea-induced increased blood pressure (BP) can be substantial (20-40 mm Hg in systolic BP and to a lesser degree in diastolic BP).

- Obesity almost always accompanies obstructive sleep apnea (OSA) and is closely correlated to a higher prevalence of hypertension.

- Correction of OSA through continuous positive airway pressure, weight loss, or surgery can markedly improve BP.

References

1. Pawar R. Blood pressure regulation and sleep apnea. A review. *Cardiovasc Rev & Rep.* 1995;16:8-24.
2. Kaplan N. *Clinical Hypertension.* Baltimore, Md: Williams & Wilkins; 1994.
3. Issa FG. Effect of clonidine in obstructive sleep apnea. *Am Rev Respir Dis.* 1992;145:435-439.

Case 12. Self-assessment questions

1. Sleep apnea is defined as respiratory cessation for 10 seconds or longer per hour for at least 10 periods during sleep.
   a. True   b. False

2. Apnea-induced increases in blood pressure (BP) tend to be greater for diastolic than systolic BP.
   a. True   b. False

3. Correction of sleep apnea can lead to a marked improvement in BP.
   a. True   b. False

Answer form on page 76.

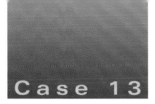

Case 13

RECALCITRANT HYPERTENSION
IN A 31-YEAR-OLD WHITE WOMAN

Patient presentation

A 31-year-old white woman presents with difficult-to-control hypertension. She has a 22-year history of diabetes mellitus of juvenile onset, and she has required insulin for the entire time. Over the last 7 years, her hypertension has become increasingly drug-resistant. She says that she carefully monitors her blood pressure (BP) at home and that it ranges from 135-145/80-90 mm Hg. She is also diligent about glycemic control, and her hemoglobin A_{1c} usually ranges between 6.5% and 7.5%. She uses little to no dietary salt. Both her mother and father have essential hypertension that requires drug therapy. She does not smoke cigarettes or drink alcohol. Her current medications include atenolol, 50 mg qd, and fosinopril, 20 mg qd.

Physical examination

On physical examination, she is 5 ft 5 in and 108 lb. BP is 144/82 mm Hg while sitting and drops to 130/70 mm Hg when standing. Her pulse is 66 beats per minute and does not change with position. Fundi show diabetic retinopathy with microaneurysms, scattered small hemorrhages, and some hardened exudates. Her chest is clear. Cardiac examination shows a regular rate and rhythm, with an S_4 gallop and a normal jugular venous pressure. Her abdomen is benign. Neurologic examination shows diminished sensation to touch in the leg and to pin prick in the midshins, bilaterally. She has 3-second capillary refill in her fingers and toes, 1+ radial pulses, and diminished dorsalis pedis pulses. There is no peripheral edema.

Laboratory evaluation

Laboratory examination shows levels of blood urea nitrogen, 26 mg/dL; total cholesterol, 188 mg/dL, with high-density lipoprotein, 26 mg/dL, and low-density lipoprotein, 136 mg/dL. Her serum creatinine level, which is normally 0.9 mg/dL, is increased to 1.4 mg/dL. Fasting glucose is 66 mg/dL. Urinalysis shows a specific gravity of 1.015, 2+ protein, 2-4 red cells, and 0-2 white cells per high-power field, and no bacteria. A 24-hour urine collection shows 690 mg of protein and 190 mEq of sodium, despite her restricted salt intake. An electrocardiogram shows normal sinus rhythm with left axis deviation and nonspecific ST-T wave changes.

What is the optimal strategy for treating this patient's condition?

Are any additional tests required?

Discussion and management

Although this patient presently has only low-grade proteinuria, such evidence clearly indicates that her diabetes has placed her at high risk for end-stage renal failure. She will require aggressive intervention to delay the rapid progression of this condition.

This patient needs both lifestyle modification and aggressive antihypertensive pharmacologic therapy, preferably with drugs that inhibit the renin-angiotensin (RA) system. She must continue to strictly monitor her glycemic control and to maintain her hemoglobin A_{1c} in its present range. According to the Diabetes Control and Complication Trial, more aggressive glycemic control can prevent progressive nephropathy.

She also needs to strictly reduce her dietary salt consumption to facilitate her BP control and to optimize the antiproteinuric effects of her antihypertensive medication, particularly if the choice is an angiotensin-converting enzyme (ACE) inhibitor. She should also begin to follow a low-saturated fat diet.

Treatment should focus on lowering her systolic BP to about 125 mm Hg, which has been found to be more satisfactory than 140 mm Hg systolic in delaying nephropathy in type 1 diabetic patients with proteinuria. At this time, the optimal antihypertensive agent for this patient would be an ACE inhibitor, which will reduce systemic pressure, glomerular capillary pressure, and transglomerular passage of albumin and proteins. The latter is an important benefit for diabetic patients, in whom glycosylated albumin is toxic to the mesangium of the kidney. Transglomerular passage of glycosylated albumin incites an inflammatory response and progressive glomerulosclerosis.

Since the patient does require a more aggressive approach to BP reduction, more than one antihypertensive agent is likely to be needed. Adding a thiazide diuretic in a low dose to the ACE inhibitor is recommended. These two agents act synergistically to lower BP. Moreover, titrating the ACE inhibitor dose upward may further lower systemic and glomerular capillary pressure. An angiotensin receptor blocker (ARB) may be used as alternate therapy. ARBs reduce BP and proteinuria to a similar degree as the ACE inhibitors. No long-term data on the use of ARBs in delaying nephropathy are yet available, but because these agents have antihypertensive and antiproteinuric properties similar to those of the ACE inhibitors, they may also delay nephropathy.

Although a β-blocker may also help lower BP in this patient, these drugs can mask symptoms of hypoglycemia, which is a particularly important factor in a patient with brittle or fluctuating glycemic control. Other vasodilators, such as calcium channel blockers and α-blockers, may also be used.

When reducing BP in diabetic patients, it is important to be mindful of an increased prevalence of orthostatic hypotension. Antihypertensive therapy may have to be tailored to fit the position (lying, sitting, standing) of the patient. Some patients require support hose to maintain BP while sitting or standing. These patients may need greater doses of medication at night when they are recumbent. Clonidine, 0.1-0.2 mg, or captopril, 12-25 mg, at bedtime can help control nocturnal BP.

Additional tests to document the cause of the patient's renal insufficiency are probably not needed. If the patient experiences incontinence or is unable to evacuate the bladder, a postvoid residual volume test or renal ultrasound may be necessary. Otherwise, the patient's changes in BP and proteinuria can be assumed to be indicative of early diabetic nephropathy.

CLINICAL PEARLS AND PITFALLS

- Because this patient has diabetes, proteinuria, and early evidence of nephropathy, her systolic blood pressure (BP) should be reduced to 125 mm Hg.

- Angiotensin-converting enzyme (ACE) inhibitors are the drugs of choice in this case. An angiotensin receptor blocker (ARB) is a suitable alternative. Clinical trials are underway to see if ARBs help delay the progression of renal disease in diabetic nephropathy.

- Reducing the patient's daily dietary salt intake (from her current 190 mEq to about 120 mEq) can substantially amplify the antihypertensive and antiproteinuric effects of the ACE inhibitor.

- Because this is a complicated case of hypertension and the patient's systolic BP should be lowered to about 125 mm Hg, two or three drugs may be required to protect her renal function. High-dose ACE inhibitors and low-dose hydrochlorothiazide, with or without a third agent, would be optimal.

Additional reading

Diabetes Control and Complications Trial Group. The effect of intensive treatment of diabetes on the development and progression of long-term complications in insulin-dependent diabetes mellitus. *N Engl J Med*. 1993;329:977-986.

Heeg JE, De Jong PE, van der Hem GK, et al. Efficacy and variability of the antiproteinuric effect of ACE inhibition by lisinopril. *Kidney Int*. 1989;36:272-279.

Lewis EJ, Hunsicker LG, Bain RP, et al. The effect of angiotensin converting enzyme inhibition on diabetic nephropathy. *N Engl J Med*. 1993;329:1456-1462.

Weir MR, Dengel DR, Behrens MT, et al. Salt-induced increases in systolic blood pressure affect renal hemodynamics and proteinuria. *Hypertension*. 1995;25:1339-1344.

Weir MR, Dworkin LD. Antihypertensive drugs, dietary salt, and renal protection: How low should you go and with which therapy? *Am J Kidney Dis*. 1998;32:1-22.

Case 13. Self-assessment questions

1. Optimal blood pressure (BP) in a patient with hypertension, insulin-dependent diabetes, and proteinuria is 125 mm Hg.
   a. True   b. False

2. Reducing dietary salt intake is crucial to potentiate the antihypertensive and antiproteinuric effects of an angiotensin-converting enzyme (ACE) inhibitor.
   a. True   b. False

3. Angiotensin receptor blockers and ACE inhibitors reduce BP and proteinuria to a similar degree.
   a. True   b. False

4. In diabetic patients with hypertension, all of the following *except* _____ delay the progression to renal disease.
   a. lowering systolic BP to 125 mm Hg
   b. strictly controlling glucose levels
   c. reducing dietary protein intake
   d. reducing saturated fat intake

Answer form on page 76.

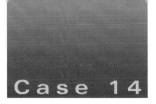

Case 14

LEFT-SIDED WEAKNESS AND SLURRED SPEECH
IN AN OLDER PATIENT

Patient presentation

A 76-year-old retired registered nurse comes to the office and describes a short episode of left-sided weakness and slurred speech. The patient has a 6-year history of hypertension, which benazepril initially controlled. Her medical records show that she suffered a similar 30-minute episode of left hemiparesis about 4 years ago. At that time, a carotid duplex study did not show any significant carotid artery disease. She was given enteric-coated aspirin, 325 mg daily.

At her current visit, her blood pressure (BP) is 180/100 mm Hg in both arms. She is given slow-release diltiazem and hydrochlorothiazide. During this visit, she experiences an episode of substernal chest pain that radiates to her back, and she is admitted to a local hospital.

Physical examination

Her BP is well controlled at 134/74 mm Hg, and she has an S_4. The rest of the cardiovascular examination is unremarkable.

Laboratory evaluation

A repeat duplex carotid scan shows no significant changes. A chest film shows mild cardiomegaly, but the mediastinum is not enlarged. A 12-lead electrocardiogram shows voltage indicative of left ventricular hypertrophy (LVH). A two-dimensional echocardiogram shows normal aortic root and confirms the presence of concentric LVH. Left ventricular ejection fraction is normal.

An abdominal sonogram shows kidneys and abdominal aorta of normal size and no gallbladder disease. Cardiac enzymes are normal, as is a dual isotope stress test. Levels of serum potassium, blood urea nitrogen, creatinine, and fasting blood sugar are normal. Other levels are: low-density lipoprotein, 185 mg/dL; high-density lipoprotein, 56 mg/dL.

Because of the presence of concentric LVH, she is given losartan, 50 mg daily, with the hydrochlorothiazide. Her BP is again taken and is 128/70 mm Hg. She is scheduled for a follow-up echocardiogram to assess the effect of losartan on her LVH.

Questions

What was the pathogenesis of left ventricular hypertrophy in this patient?

On what basis should therapy be chosen?

Discussion and management

In this patient, the left ventricle adapted to sustained arterial hypertension by becoming concentrically hypertrophic. This process is rather complex because of the concomitant effect of volume load, the myocardial inotropic state, and nonhemodynamic factors.

In an echocardiographic study of 165 patients with untreated hypertension, 52% had normal left ventricular mass index and normal left relative wall thickness.[1] Of the remaining patients, 27% showed concentric remodeling (normal left ventricular mass with increased relative wall thickness) and 8% showed typical hypertensive concentric hypertrophy (increased left ventricular mass with increased relative wall thickness). These classifications were based on left ventricular geometric patterns.

In addition, patients with increased ventricular mass had a higher incidence of morbid events (death, myocardial infarct, stroke, angina, heart failure).[2] This was true despite the fact that most of these patients were taking antihypertensive medication. Patients with concentric LVH had increased carotid arterial wall thickness and increased plaque formation.[3]

Even in the absence of coronary artery disease, echocardiographic LVH is significantly associated with increased frequency and complexity of ventricular arrhythmias. This observation has established LVH as an independent risk factor for sudden cardiac death.[4,5]

Classifying LVH by geometric patterns is helpful in selecting appropriate antihypertensive therapy.[6] Patients with normal left ventricular geometry can be treated nonpharmacologically, with weight control, alcohol avoidance, and caloric restriction. Those with concentric left ventricular remodeling due to elevated peripheral resistance may benefit from peripheral vasodilators. In eccentric LVH, a diuretic combined with an angiotensin-converting enzyme (ACE) inhibitor is the treatment of choice. In patients with concentric LVH, drugs that normalize peripheral resistance, induce regression of LVH, and reduce volume load are indicated. Angiotensin receptor blockers (ARBS) and ACE inhibitors in combination with diuretics or β-blockers are the best treatment in these patients with high cardiovascular risks. ARBs and ACE inhibitors have similar efficacy; ARBs may regress LVH sooner and to a greater degree than ACE inhibitors.

CLINICAL PEARLS AND PITFALLS

- Left ventricular hypertrophy (LVH) is an independent risk factor for sudden cardiac death because of its association with ventricular arrhythmias.

- Drugs that decrease peripheral vascular resistance can reduce concentric LVH.

- Hypertensive patients with normal left ventricular geometry can be treated nonpharmacologically with weight control and alcohol avoidance.

References

1. Ganau A, Devereux RB, Roman MJ, et al. Patterns of left ventricular hypertrophy and geometric remodeling in essential hypertension. *J Am Coll Cardiol.* 1992;19:1550-1558.
2. Koren MJ, Devereux RB, Casale PN, et al. Relation of left ventricular mass and geometry to morbidity and mortality in uncomplicated essential hypertension. *Ann Intern Med.* 1991;114:345-352.
3. Roman MJ, Pickering TG, Schwartz JE, et al. Relation of arterial structure and function to left ventricular geometric patterns in hypertensive adults. *J Am Coll Cardiol.* 1996;28:751-756.
4. Levy D, Anderson K, Savage DD, et al. Risk of ventricular arrhythmias in left ventricular hypertrophy: The Framingham Heart Study. *Am J Cardiol.* 1987;60:560-565.
5. Ghali JK, Kadakia S, Cooper RS, et al. Impact of left ventricular hypertrophy on ventricular arrhythmias in the absence of coronary artery disease. *J Am Coll Cardiol.* 1991;17:1277-1282.
6. Ganau A, Devereux RB. Ventricular patterns in hypertensive patients: Pathogenesis, treatment, and prognosis. *Prim Cardiol.* 1994;20:19-27.

Case 14. Self-assessment questions

1. Left ventricular hypertrophy (LVH) is a risk factor for sudden cardiac death only because of its association with coronary artery disease.
   a. True   b. False

2. Drugs that increase peripheral vascular resistance can reverse LVH.
   a. True   b. False

3. Drugs that decrease peripheral vascular resistance can reverse concentric LVH.
   a. True   b. False

Answer form on page 76.

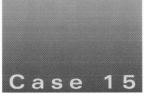

Case 15

PERFUSE PERSPIRATION, SHORTNESS OF BREATH, AND CHEST PRESSURE IN AN AFRICAN-AMERICAN MAN

Patient presentation

A 53-year-old African-American man presents with perfuse perspiration, shortness of breath, and mild pressure in his chest associated with exertion. He says these symptoms began about 2 weeks earlier. He has a 3-year history of type 2 diabetes mellitus, and he has nonnephrotic-range proteinuria. His hypertension was diagnosed 2 years ago. He does not visit a physician regularly.

His medications include 70/30 insulin, 50 units, taken subcutaneously every morning; NPH insulin, 30 units, taken subcutaneously in the evening; and lisinopril, 5 mg, taken once daily. He has no known drug allergies. His family history is remarkable for type 2 diabetes in his mother and maternal grandfather, coronary artery disease in his mother at the age of 65 years, and hyperthyroidism in his sister. He drinks alcohol socially and denies tobacco use.

Physical examination

On physical examination, pulse is 76 beats per minute, blood pressure (BP), 170/92 mm Hg in the right arm and 174/90 mm Hg in the left arm. He is moderately obese, with central adiposity. His body mass index is 32. A head and neck examination is remarkable for grade 2 hypertensive changes and background diabetic retinopathy. Vertical ear lobe creases and bilateral carotid bruits are noted. There is no jugular venous distention. On cardiac examination, an S_4 is present. The point of maximal impulse is laterally displaced and sustained. There are no abdominal bruits. He has decreased vibratory sense in his bilateral lower extremities, diminished pedal pulses, and no hair on the lower extremities.

Laboratory evaluation

Laboratory studies show the following levels: creatinine, 2.0 mg/dL; total cholesterol, 327 mg/dL; triglycerides, 302 mg/dL; high-density lipoprotein, 39 mg/dL; low-density lipoprotein (LDL), 228 mg/dL; glycosylated hemoglobin, 9.7 g/dL.

Question

How should this patient be managed?

Discussion and management

This patient has several comorbid conditions that must be managed. He has complications of both diabetes and hypertension, as evidenced in clinical findings of retinopathy, nephropathy, and cardiomyopathy. The presence of typical angina with multiple risk factors confirms coronary artery disease, although concurrent small vessel disease cannot be excluded.

Aspirin and antianginal therapy should be initiated immediately. Work-up should begin with a coronary angiogram, which most authorities would recommend for a patient this age with unstable angina. Although this procedure places him at high risk for worsening nephropathy, minimizing the dye load and hydrating aggressively with diuretic therapy should reduce this risk.

Choice of medication to control his BP will depend on whether catheterization findings reveal a need for revascularization or the presence of a significant diastolic or systolic dysfunction. Complicating antihypertensive medication choices and management issues even more are his nephropathy, diabetes, and hyperlipidemia.

Given his eye ground findings, his nephropathy is likely secondary to both glomerulosclerosis (secondary to his diabetes) and nephrosclerosis (secondary to his hypertension). The possibility of atherosclerotic renal artery stenosis or angiotensin-converting enzyme (ACE) inhibition must also be considered as a cause for his elevated creatinine level. Moreover, a review of his recent blood urea nitrogen and creatinine levels would help determine if work-up is indicated. Because he has diabetes, the possibility of type IV renal tubular acidosis/hyporeninemic-hypoaldosteronism should also be considered.

To further complicate the management of this patient, his severe hyperlipidemia must be a factor in the choice of hypertensive medications. Some agents, such as high-dose diuretics, could adversely affect lipid levels, while others, such as α-blockers and ACE inhibitors, could have more favorable effects.

An angiotensin receptor blocker (ARB) would also be a reasonable choice in that preliminary data suggest that ARBs have cardioprotective and renoprotective effects similar to those of ACE inhibitors. ARBs may also be used in combination therapy.

Aggressive diabetes management with dietary therapy and oral agents, such as metformin, troglitazone, or sulfonylureas, should be initiated to lower his insulin requirements. Although control of blood sugars should improve his lipid values, a hydroxymethylglutaryl coenzyme A reductase inhibitor will most likely also be needed to lower LDL-cholesterol levels to under 100 mg/dL. These measures have the potential to arrest or even reverse atherosclerosis in this patient.

CLINICAL PEARLS AND PITFALLS

- In the setting of hypertension, diabetes, hyperlipidemia, and typical angina, urgent aggressive work-up and therapy for coronary artery disease are indicated.
- Acute changes in renal function in a patient with hypertension and diabetes warrant consideration of work-up for renal artery stenosis.
- Hyperlipidemia can complicate the choice of medications for management of both hypertension and diabetes mellitus.
- Normalizing blood sugar can help in improving lipid values in poorly controlled diabetes. This measure used in combination with newer drops that can lower insulin levels should help slow—or possibly reverse—atherosclerosis.

Additional reading

The Joint Committee on Prevention, Detection, Evaluation and Treatment of High Blood Pressure. The Sixth Report of the Joint Committee on Prevention, Detection, Evaluation, and Treatment of High Blood Pressure. *Arch Intern Med.* 1997;157:2413-2445.

Sowers JR. Impact of lipid and ACE inhibitor therapy on cardiovascular disease and metabolic abnormalities in the diabetic and hypertensive patient. *J Hum Hypertens.* 1997;11:9-16.

Steinberg HO, Chaker H, Leaming R, et al. Obesity/insulin resistance is associated with endothelial dysfunction. Implications for the syndrome of insulin resistance. *J Clin Invest.* 1996;97:2601-2610.

Case 15. Self-assessment questions

1. High-dose diuretics should be used routinely in patients who have diabetes, hypertension, and hyperlipidemia.
   a. True   b. False

2. In the setting of hypertension and diabetes, _____ can cause azotemia.
   a. nephrosclerosis
   b. glomerulosclerosis
   c. renal artery stenosis
   d. All of the above

3. Troglitazone is a good choice for managing diabetes, because it raises insulin levels.
   a. True   b. False

4. In type 2 diabetic patients with hypertension and coronary artery disease, _____.
   a. low-density lipoprotein levels should be lowered to under 100 mg/dL
   b. insulin is always the drug of choice to control blood sugar
   c. β-blockers are contraindicated
   d. All of the above

Answer form on page 76.

Evaluation

We would like your opinion regarding this and future activities. Please circle the appropriate answers, and return this evaluation with your CME registration (page 75) and self-assessment answer forms (page 76).

1. On the whole, how do you rate the information in this activity?
   a. Excellent   c. Fair
   b. Good   d. Poor

2. Please describe one way that you plan to change the management of hypertension in your practice after participating in this activity.
   _____
   _____
   _____

3. Do you have any recommendations for improving this activity?
   a. Yes   b. No
   Comments_____
   _____
   _____

4. Were any portions of this activity unsatisfactory or inappropriate?
   a. Yes   b. No
   If so, which? _____
   _____
   _____

5. Please rate this activity with regard to fair balance, scientific rigor, and avoidance of commercial bias.
   a. Excellent   c. Fair
   b. Good   d. Poor

6. Please indicate the length of time it took you to complete this activity, including the self-assessment questions and this evaluation.
   a. Less than 60 minutes
   b. 60 to 80 minutes
   c. 80 to 100 minutes
   d. 100 to 120 minutes
   e. More than 120 minutes

In the following, please indicate how relevant the activity content was to each learning objective.

7. Objective 1
   a. Completely   b. Partially   c. Not at all

8. Objective 2
   a. Completely   b. Partially   c. Not at all

9. Objective 3
   a. Completely   b. Partially   c. Not at all

10. Objective 4
   a. Completely   b. Partially   c. Not at all

11. Objective 5
   a. Completely   b. Partially   c. Not at all

In the following, please indicate how well you achieved the stated learning objective after completing this activity.

12. Objective 1
   a. Completely   b. Partially   c. Not at all

13. Objective 2
   a. Completely   b. Partially   c. Not at all

14. Objective 3
   a. Completely   b. Partially   c. Not at all

15. Objective 4
   a. Completely   b. Partially   c. Not at all

16. Objective 5
   a. Completely   b. Partially   c. Not at all

CME registration form
Diagnosing hypertension

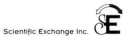
Scientific Exchange Inc.

Date   Social Security number

☐☐ / ☐☐ / ☐☐☐☐
Month   Day   Year

☐☐☐ - ☐☐ - ☐☐☐☐

Name

☐☐☐☐☐☐☐☐☐☐☐☐☐☐☐☐   ☐
First   MI

☐☐☐☐☐☐☐☐☐☐☐☐☐☐☐☐☐
Last

Home address

☐☐☐☐☐☐☐☐☐☐☐☐☐☐☐☐☐
Street

☐☐☐☐☐☐☐☐☐☐☐☐☐☐☐☐☐

☐☐☐☐☐☐☐☐☐☐☐☐☐   ☐☐   ☐☐☐☐☐
City   State   Zip

Daytime phone number

☐☐☐ - ☐☐☐ - ☐☐☐☐

To request Continuing Medical Education credit:

Processing
You may submit this completed form in one of three ways.

1. *Fax* to (516) 563-1907, 24 hours a day, 7 days a week.
2. *Mail* to Program Management Services, Inc., PO Box 490, East Islip, NY 11730.
3. *Telephone* 1-800-405-2347, 10 AM to 5 PM EST, Monday through Friday.
   Please have your credit card handy.

Processing times
Fax—7 days; mail—2-4 weeks; telephone—4 days

Payment information
The processing fee is $10.00. If your payment is by check, please make payable to Program Management Services, Inc. If by credit card, please complete the following:

Credit card   ☐ Visa   ☐ MasterCard   ☐ American Express   Expiration date ____ / ____

Credit card number ☐☐☐☐☐☐☐☐☐☐☐☐☐☐☐☐

Authorized signature _____

Answer form: Self-assessment questions

For each question, choose the best answer and place an x through that box. If you change an answer, be sure to erase completely. Mark only one answer for each question.

Case 1   1. [a] [b]
         2. [a] [b]
         3. [a] [b] [c] [d]
         4. [a] [b]

Case 6   1. [a] [b]
         2. [a] [b]
         3. [a] [b] [c] [d]

Case 11 1. [a] [b] [c] [d] [e]
         2. [a] [b] [c] [d] [e]
         3. [a] [b] [c] [d] [e]
         4. [a] [b] [c] [d] [e]

Case 2   1. [a] [b] [c] [d] [e]
         2. [a] [b]
         3. [a] [b]
         4. [a] [b]

Case 7   1. [a] [b]
         2. [a] [b]
         3. [a] [b]
         4. [a] [b]

Case 12 1. [a] [b]
         2. [a] [b]
         3. [a] [b]

Case 3   1. [a] [b] [c] [d] [e]
         2. [a] [b] [c] [d] [e]
         3. [a] [b] [c] [d]
         4. [a] [b] [c] [d] [e]

Case 8   1. [a] [b] [c] [d] [e]
         2. [a] [b] [c] [d]
         3. [a] [b] [c] [d] [e]
         4. [a] [b] [c] [d] [e]

Case 13 1. [a] [b]
         2. [a] [b]
         3. [a] [b]
         4. [a] [b] [c] [d]

Case 4   1. [a] [b] [c] [d]
         2. [a] [b]
         3. [a] [b]
         4. [a] [b] [c] [d]

Case 9   1. [a] [b]
         2. [a] [b]
         3. [a] [b] [c] [d]

Case 14 1. [a] [b]
         2. [a] [b]
         3. [a] [b]

Case 5   1. [a] [b]
         2. [a] [b]
         3. [a] [b] [c] [d]

Case 10 1. [a] [b]
         2. [a] [b]
         3. [a] [b]

Case 15 1. [a] [b]
         2. [a] [b] [c] [d]
         3. [a] [b]
         4. [a] [b] [c] [d]

I am a ___ physician ___ nonphysician.

I certify that I have completed this activity as designed.

Signature_____